# The Invisible Prison

# The
# Invisible
# Prison

*A HANDBOOK FOR MULTIPLE*
*CHEMICAL SENSITIVITY*

EVELYN TODD

Matador
9 Priory Business Park
Kibworth Beauchamp
Leicestershire LE8 0RX, UK
Tel: (+44) 116 279 2299
Fax: (+44) 116 279 2277
Email: books@troubador.co.uk
Web: www.troubador.co.uk/matador

ISBN 978 1784621 773

British Library Cataloguing in Publication Data.
A catalogue record for this book is available from the British Library.

Printed and bound in the UK by TJ International, Padstow, Cornwall
Typeset in Aldine by Troubador Publishing Ltd

**Matador** is an imprint of Troubador Publishing Ltd

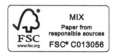

The cover picture is of a solarium in the Valley Gardens, Harrogate. It can be taken as symbolic of life with MCS – inside a drab room but with attractive, enticing possibilities outside that cannot be reached because there are bars. Hopefully, some day and with luck perhaps, it may be possible to climb over those bars.

# CONTENTS

Introduction                                                    xi

SECTION A: APPROACH TO THE PROBLEM  1
How to use this book – special glossary – the
problem – what is Multiple Chemical
Sensitivity? – possible causes – disbelief and
disbelievers – the psychological theory – has
the answer to all this been found? – summary
definition of MCS – examples of the
symptoms – results of MCS – treatment –
the role of health professionals.

SECTION B : CHEMICALS IN THE
ENVIRONMENT – PAST AND PRESENT       25
Some chemical substances commonly at fault
in MCS – formaldehyde – bronopol-
methanol- air fresheners – perfumes – a
diversion into the past – lead – mercury –
arsenic – air pollution – asbestos – the modern
toxic soup – modern pollutants which can
cause problems – ozone – formaldehyde –
insecticides – pesticides – mercury now –
volatile organic compounds – polychlorinated
biphenyls – phthalates – surfactants – dioxins
– indoor pollution – endnote.

SECTION C: THOSE AFFECTED SPEAK          51

SECTION D: COPING WITH THE
CONDITION                                75

Warning – adjustment – making a start – the articulate advocate – a medallion-knowing your enemies – avoidance and protection – cutting down your chemical burden – a safe home – toilet preparations-cosmetics – visitors and callers – cleaning without harmful chemicals – dishwashing – laundry – dry cleaning – bathrooms and shower cubicles – lessening soiling.

Ventilation – redecorating – choosing a home or making do with what we have – outgassing.

General health – food – teeth – allergies and intolerances – general comments on diet – cooking – food preparation – food storage – saucepans etc. – dietary supplements – water and beverages – soft drinks and alcohol.

Candida – brain fog and lethargy – Irritable bowel syndrome – nasal blockage

Going out and exercise – going on holiday – travel – air conditioning.

Other people –doctors–dentists–hospitals

Rest and sleep – challenges – pushing ones boundaries – electrical sensitivity

The spiritual dimension.

SUMMARY                          144

FURTHER READING                  149

USEFUL ADDRESSES                 151

GLOSSARY                         154

INDEX                            159

# INTRODUCTION

The aim of this book is threefold: firstly, to provide as much information and advice as I can, for those with Multiple Chemical Sensitivity, on how to manage their condition; secondly, to raise awareness of, and in so doing explain, Multiple Chemical Sensitivity to any who come into contact with them and to describe the problems it poses to the sufferers and their families in their daily existence and hence their needs.

As, to my knowledge, nothing of this sort has been written on this side of the Atlantic, I hope to raise awareness of the condition especially among health professionals for whom this is paramount. I hope they will consent to read this – at least the salient parts of it. For them it should make easy reading. Hopefully it will not be long before the condition is recognised as a physical illness in this country, as it is in others in the developed world, which is my third aim.

I have collected as much information and advice about the condition, from now on sometimes referred to as MCS, as I have been able. I embarked on talking on the telephone to as many people as I could who suffer from MCS. It had to be by phone or email because for us it is difficult, sometimes it is impossible, to travel, visit other people's homes or receive visitors.

Therefore, this has had to be a desktop study.

Very early on in my research it became apparent that I must try to make our common plight public as soon as possible. Unlike most other conditions it is important that everyone coming near someone with MCS understands, at least roughly, what their problem is. For example, hopefully, to stop the teenager in their presence suddenly bringing out a spray and spraying themself with perfume. Also, that those enquiries about the use of air fresheners or contents of food are honestly answered.

At the outset I had decided to discount any revelations that seemed to carry any suggestion whatever of exaggeration or theatricality or for any other reason caused me to doubt their validity. Believe me, my professional experience has left me prone to be both dubious and suspicious of much I am told. But, to date, I have found none that fits those categories in those who truly have the condition. There are many persons who find themselves suffering from a sensitivity to one or two particular chemicals but they are not considered here. With us multiple means multiple.

I have been surprised at the factual and calm manner by which people I contacted related to me serious daily difficulties they were, and still will be, encountering. In short I have been impressed by their courage and stoicism. However, most of those I contacted had at one time or other volunteered to give advice and support to other sufferers. This makes them an untypical sample, leaving me to fear that there is a hidden unknown number out there, perplexed and unaware how to cope.

At the time of writing, although Multiple Chemical Sensitivity is recognised as a serious illness in Germany, Denmark, Austria, Luxembourg, Japan, Canada and the USA, it is not recognised in the UK. Why, I ask? As it is not a recognised condition we have to pay Value Added Tax on items such as the necessary vapour masks which normally, as they are for medical use, we should not. Amongst all our other problems this is an additional unkindness. Recently I was charged two pounds each Value Added Tax on the carbon filters I need to protect me in my own home. Why is Britain lagging behind in recognition?

The prevalence of the condition in this country as it is not an "official illness" is not known. Figures I have seen have been 0.5% Germany, 3.7% Sweden, 3.8% Japan and 3.9% USA respectively for the severest form whilst figures given for a more moderate varied between 9% and 33%. As I have indicated there are large numbers of people who find that one or more chemicals that they encounter in their daily life make them unwell but the problem can be overcome perhaps by an analgesic or an inhaler. But with Multiple Chemical Sensitivity numerous chemicals are involved and the symptoms are severe and disabling.

Some people, as I was for many years, and even their doctors, will be unaware that chemical pollution causes their symptoms. To other patients it has become all too obvious but there may be little advice available to them. We find ourselves living in an insecure no-man's-land.

Some professionals acknowledge the existence of our condition but many do not. Most have little knowledge or understanding of it. This is most unfortunate, can cause us much discomfort and could prove dangerous. Any facilities or a protocol necessary for our care when in hospital, if they do exist in this country, must be extremely rare.

Some years ago I walked up to the reception desk in Moorfields Eye Hospital in London. I merely had to repeat the diagnosis made by my GP of a suspected detached retina and everything was immediately set in motion. I was dealt with swiftly and efficiently and later that morning emerged outside once again, clutching a card for a follow-up appointment. Mentioning the letters MCS should also be met with equal understanding.

Currently most MCS sufferers, whatever other condition takes them to a hospital, will have to explain MCS and negotiate to be protected from the ambient gases, other patient perfumes, etc., request the concessions to diet and other things. As well as this, they also hope to describe the problem that has brought them there. They will also hope that admitting to MCS will not stop their other symptoms being taken seriously.

At a time when they are at their most anxious and vulnerable, some staff, being ignorant of the condition, are as likely to be impatient and sceptical as they are to be understanding. Thus, as well as suffering from their presenting condition, the patient is likely to suffer complications they could have been protected from.

This could be dangerous. My personal experience has been that health professionals are kind and eager to do their best but difficulties arise because, mostly, they have no knowledge of the condition. I believe that the harm and discomforts I have suffered over the years in various places have been purely the result of ignorance.

This is not a medical text. I do not presume to know anything about the diagnosis and treatment of the condition other than suggestions I have met, briefly, in my researches. I set out to inform patients on how to cope with their condition on a day-to-day basis and to explain their problems to their relatives and friends and importantly to the health professionals whom they will encounter.

MCS has been described as a devastating and isolating illness and I would add an expensive one as well. Illnesses tend to cause expense but mostly the items purchased can be of use. But as well as paying Value Added Tax, that if their medical needs were accepted they would be exempt from, most sufferers will have bought items in the hope that they can be of use only to find they cannot tolerate the presence of their purchase. Commonly, only the most costly is suitable. An item minus an ingredient is usually more expensive than with it. Also there is the risk from the spurious claims from some alternative medicine practitioners and vendors. Although it is mandatory for food producers to state changes in ingredients on labels this does not apply to other manufacturers. So it seems frequent that buying an article, for example soap, previously found to be safe, results in disappointment because a new chemical perfume has been added making it unusable.

For some this text may seem over inclusive and at times repetitive. But my experience with the general public is that firstly even the most well-informed individuals have some gaps and secondly, when putting over any concept, repetition aids memory. What seems self-evident to some will be news to others. So please bear with me those who find this patronising. It is not intended to be.

In writing this I am not seeking sympathy for us but I am seeking to engender understanding and belief. Although at present there seems to be no cure for this condition, which is chronic and can be progressive, if we are treated with empathy and kindness it certainly lightens our burden.

Logically I will describe the condition first then look at chemicals in the environment, past and present. Next is a section on experiencing MCS before I go on to advise those with MCS on how they may best live with it. But I must stress this is advice in generality. It cannot be applicable or feasible to everyone. Above all some suggestions MAY NOT BE SAFE for some and I cannot take any responsibility for any adverse outcome. Those following my suggestions must do so at their own risk and must make their own assessment for their own safety. Check with your doctor or another health professional, if you can, about things that you are not sure of or be prepared to follow the old adage, "If in doubt leave it out".

# APPROACH TO THE PROBLEM

## EVERYONE

Please look at the SPECIAL GLOSSARY first. Most references are added in italics at the end of the passage. For aid in cross referencing whilst using the book there are comprehensive contents and index sections. Spaces in the text will allow users to add their own notes and comments.

## SUFFERERS FROM MCS

You may want to go straight to Section D on Coping with the Condition but please read the opening paragraph before you dip into the text. Do not be put off by the vastness of the advice offered. Some will not be appropriate. Some will not be possible. Some will seem too difficult. But do not give up. Look at it and select what you can easily do. Later, take on some of the difficult and leave the seemingly impossible till last as some of it may become possible in the fullness of time.

Everyone will not be able to do everything, I do not myself. But my experience leads me to believe that a period of some months of strict avoidance of all chemicals possible to avoid, as well as, importantly, those known to cause problems, is beneficial. After this, one can perhaps relax a little. My advice may seem like pie in the sky to some but believe me I do know what it is like to stand with a trolley at the entrance to a supermarket and wonder how on earth I will summon up enough energy to push it to the other end.

The main aim will be to lighten the chemical burden on your body. This is not an offer of cure but some hints on coping and achieving a more comfortable existence. Hopefully it will also lessen the severity of symptoms and slow the progress of the condition. But, I repeat, follow the advice after due thinking if it is safe for you and go ahead with care at your own responsibility. Improvement is unlikely to come overnight but hopefully there will be some, although it may take many months.

## RELATIVES, FRIENDS AND HEALTH PROFESSIONALS

I suggest that you start reading at the beginning. The advice section will be less relevant to you but if you read the whole book it will increase your understanding and empathy for MCS sufferers. As Nurse Tutor I used to encourage my students to read books written by patients about their experience of their illness. It results in a more rounded view of the patient, aids rapport and may even explain sometimes otherwise puzzling behaviour. Therefore I hope you will read sections C and D.

Nurses – The patient will depend on you to protect them from the chemicals that harm them. You will need to arrange that inpatients are nursed in a safe environment. This, of course, can only be satisfactorily achieved by the use of a single room with the door clearly labelled prohibiting the entry of everyone until vetted by you as not carrying vapours on their person. Every hospital should have a protocol for the care of MCS patients and all staff should know of it. Please see also THE ROLE OF HEALTH PROFESSIONALS.

# SPECIAL GLOSSARY

Below are the meanings of terms as used in this text. They may have other meanings elsewhere. A more general glossary will be found at the end of the document.

ALLERGEN – That which causes an adverse reaction as above.

ALLERGY – A blanket term for reacting adversely to something not normally reacted against or reacted to when in smaller amounts than would normally be expected. For convenience I may not differentiate between allergy, sensitivity or intolerance.

BACKGROUND POLLUTION – Vapours and dusts which exist in the air constantly and which can emanate from natural occurrences like volcanoes and forest fires but now come predominantly from modern sources such as industry and vehicle emissions.

BRAIN FOG – Clarity of thought is lost. Thus the performing of simple calculations accurately is impeded, decisions on a course of action are difficult and the patient, having waited in a polluted waiting room, finds describing their symptoms clearly to a physician problematical.

DISBELIEVER – Someone who either denies that the condition exists or denies that it has a physiological origin.

DISSEMINATOR – A person whose heavy use of personal care items such as deodorants, aftershave and perfume, results in a heavy load of artificial chemical vapours on the air around them, perhaps stretching to a number of metres, even outdoors. The air can even remain polluted when they have reached some distance away. Indoors, their pollution remains long after they have left a room as it can cling to soft furnishings and remain in air pockets. To MCS sufferers, who can become ill in the presence of persons who make only moderate use of personal toilet preparations, these persons are a decided menace. The perfume from the detergents and fabric conditioners they use may also be adding to the total load that this person disseminates.

INCITANT – That which will cause a symptom to occur.

OUTGASSING – The process of items giving off chemical vapours, generally doing so less over the passage of time. Sometimes the process can be speeded up. Those with MCS need to leave new things somewhere away from their living areas to outgas before they are safe for use.

PASS OUT – The end stage of some reactions to chemicals when the patient falls irresistibly into a deep sleep for some time. On waking, recovery is likely to have started.

## THE PROBLEM

Our bodies are made up of an assortment of chemicals and sceptics are eager to point this out. We need a regular intake of some chemicals to remain healthy, even to stay alive. But those same chemicals, for example, zinc, which is needed for many body processes, can be toxic if taken in excess: as a woman who made marmalade in a zinc-lined bucket discovered. The acid in the oranges caused the zinc to leach into the contents of the bucket and those who ate the marmalade suffered poisoning. But MCS is not like having been poisoned and then having recovered. Neither is it an allergy but it is similar in that exposures to small amounts can result in, sometimes violent, responses each time they happen.

There are many chemicals in our modern environment. We are now exposed to many more man-made chemicals than humans have ever been in the whole of history. Mostly these are believed to be at a level low enough for them to be harmless. However, some of us are made ill by these sometimes minute amounts of chemicals that we encounter. Sometimes, I believe, there are very small traces indeed. It is now very common to be sensitive to some chemical or other; such as rashes from detergents, headaches from fresh paint, asthma from perfume. But some people are sensitive to so many, or react so severely, that this becomes a major impediment to daily living. For some it can even be life threatening. It is likely that in some situations airborne chemicals can combine producing problems that alone they might not cause. Unaware to the individual, chemicals can enter the body through the mouth in food, water or even medicines and by contamination of the hands. They can be breathed in and they are sometimes absorbed through the skin. For many who are affected it results in major employment, financial, housing, health and social consequences.

## SO WHAT IS MULTIPLE CHEMICAL SENSITIVITY?

It is a little understood, often progressive, condition which results in the sufferer reacting adversely to chemicals encountered in the environment when they are at levels not affecting the rest of the community or that had not affected them previously. It was once called "allergy to the twentieth century". Perhaps TILT – Toxicant Induced Loss of Tolerance – is a preferable name.

Frequently it manifests itself first after a period of illness, often a viral one, or other stress. Previously there will have been a massive exposure to a chemical, or a long exposure at a lower level, commonly in gaseous form. Once sensitised the individual often becomes sensitive to other chemicals. Chemicals normally used in the home are major hazards. Daily life becomes a constant problem because even at home it is difficult to avoid these incitants as callers, for example even paramedics called to another member of the family, can bring vapours with them. The opening of a parcel can release harmful vapours or gases can waft through a window from a neighbour's washing line.

An example of a victim is a draughtsman who was exposed to excessive quantities of ammonia at work. Starting with "flu like" symptoms he became ill when encountering paint, creosote, crop spray, household polishes and sheep dip and of course even the smell of women's perfume affected him. He had become so ill that he had become housebound. His symptoms included chest pains and respiratory problems.

Although it is good advice in general to have a positive attitude and to strive for a normal way of life, severity of symptoms often prevents this. So, like this man, the individual becomes housebound or at best lives an extremely restricted life. Socially isolated the sufferer may also become estranged from their spouse or other members of family too because they cannot understand the condition or cannot tolerate the restriction it puts upon them. Fatigue, lethargy and brain fog can make daily activity difficult and can be symptoms which others find hard to understand. For those unable to work there are financial problems.

The process by which the symptoms arise seems complicated. It is thought that there is another factor, or factors, probably in the atmosphere, besides the recognised incitants that are involved and that it is not primarily due to involvement of the nose. My personal experience has been that I have recovered from moderate reactions in the following places; the Louvre in Paris, the Royal Festival Hall in London and a local supermarket. The common factor between all these is air conditioning. Even being in a car with the air conditioning running can sometimes bring some relief. It is important to get away from an incitant as soon as possible but going outdoors to safety does not stop a reaction that has begun although, hopefully, it may make it less severe.

The conditions Myalgic Encephalomyelitis and Fibromyalgia have some similarity to MCS in that sufferers are sensitive to chemicals and one of these may coexist with it. It is also said that Porphyria frequently coexists with MCS. Food allergies, other allergies and intolerances are very common as is the overgrowth of candida. Candida may have a causative role and it can affect many systems of the body, particularly the endocrine system. Frequently other, often major, medical conditions coexist with MCS.

Although it is unknown how many people are affected by this condition in the UK it is believed that the number is growing. Women seem to be affected in greater numbers than men possibly because they are at home for longer periods and thus more exposed to indoor pollutants, particularly cleaning materials. Sometimes a person with MCS comes from a family with a tendency to allergies but as that situation is so common it may not be relevant. But other than these it seems that no type of individual is more likely to succumb than any other.

A study in south eastern USA in 2004 reported that sensitivity was more common in females but otherwise experienced by both sexes of a variety of ages and educational levels. The condition mostly manifests itself first in adulthood and may worsen with age. Some say we have a particularly good sense of smell. But this may be that result of our efforts to live in a pure environment leaves us with our natural sense of smell when it may have become blunted in others by over exposure. I have frequently detected gas leaks that others could not sense; even to being specifically contacted by a gas board engineer who thanked me for so accurately pin pointing an outdoor leak for him. I was interested to learn that the Mau Mau in Kenya in the 1950s frequently evaded the British soldiers who were seeking them out because not only could they hear them, they could also smell the British coming. Although male toilet preparations were far more restricted in those days cigarette smoking was considered a norm. The nasal senses of the Mau Mau had presumably not been blunted by similar practices.

## POSSIBLE CAUSES

Some authorities believe that the condition is a result of the detoxification pathways of the body having been overwhelmed by environmental assaults. Others feel that there is some deficiency in the enzyme systems. My personal experience and recent reading would make me opt for the former. But perhaps it is a chicken and egg situation. But as I am not qualified to judge I will say no more other than to comment that there seems to be, sometimes, an unfortunate tendency to consider those who succumb to the condition to be inferior specimens. Individuals have varying susceptibilities. My husband was once overwhelmed by "hay fever" whilst I, in the same environment, was completely unaffected. Why should reacting to pollens be acceptable but chemicals not? It may be noted that since moving from London my husband has become markedly better from the condition.

It is known that some chemicals, for example, lead, once absorbed never get broken down or excreted from the body.

## DISBELIEF AND DISBELIEVERS

As well as the problems resulting from the symptoms of this condition those who have been smitten with it have to contend with those who do not believe it exists. With other conditions, that mostly will not matter but those with MCS depend on the cooperation of those around them not to do anything that will cause them to become ill so it becomes a problem. In reality professed disbelief by those close to an individual may more likely be denial.

Yes, MCS is difficult to understand but so are many modern illnesses. When one leaves the realms of infection and malnutrition, which were the models for disease in past times, those with little knowledge of physiology may find many conditions incomprehensible but hopefully, still accept that the individuals are sick. Our experience suggests a new mechanism or theory of disease – an initial salient exposure with thereafter a reaction to well tolerated substances. It has been said, "The industrial age has brought about exposures to a steady concentration of substances for which our biological evolution did not prepare us".

No doubt a psychological paper could be written on denial in our situation. But perhaps it is sufficient to say that everyone has their own fears and anxieties. Some may feel that their relative is letting the side down by professing to a strange and chronic illness. Others, full of concern and sympathy, just cannot bear to see it happening to a loved one or are fearful of the outcome. Others may have less altruistic agendas.

The allergic-like reaction of sufferers is hard to accept for those who associate such responses with protein although there has been some suggestion that in our case a chemical has bonded with a protein. Others of this group argue from the point of view that as we are built up of chemicals, how can we be sensitive to them? Hopefully they do not, on other occasions, complain that something or other, for example fresh paint, gives them a headache! It is good to be sceptical about new ideas and one can sympathise when it is health professionals who are being dubious of a condition not recognised in this country and about which they have not been taught. Also the amount of self diagnosis and self identification of incitants, that out of necessity occurs, can arouse suspicions in those unaware of the reality of the condition. But it is disbelief in this group that can be so devastating to us.

I object strongly to the move to call the condition "Idiopathic Environmental Illness" as if there was no obvious external cause. It is quite obvious that there are plenty of chemicals around us. As I have said not everyone becomes ill but neither does everyone become affected when the pollen count becomes high. Nevertheless pollen is accepted as a cause of rhinitis.

*Helke Ferrie,* (KOS Publishing, 1997), Beech Gove Road, Ontario LON 1AD
*Email: Helke@inetonic.com*

## THE "PSYCHOLOGICAL" THEORY

*"Difficulty lies, not in new ideas but in escaping
from the old ones."*
*Maynard Keynes*

This is a leviathan that still needs to be slain although, having had its heyday in the middle of the last century, one would have hoped that by now it would be getting too elderly and infirm to signify. I admit to feeling particularly militant against it because of the affect it has had on my self esteem for most of my life.

A psychological explanation is a soft and convenient theory that can be easily wrapped around any problem that otherwise has no obvious explanation. It was applied frequently to illnesses in the 1950s and 1960s; sometimes, in my own observation, with fatal results. Sadly it is still around. Sigmund Freud led doctors to believe that women were likely to consult them over conditions with no physical base and even worse perhaps, fall in love with them, doctors all being male in those days, and make themselves nuisances. This has made difficulties over conditions where the sufferers are all mainly women; even for females who are doctors themselves. The mind and body are inextricably linked.

Whether an individual succumbs to a particular illness can depend on a single factor or many working together. The intangibles that give us a sense of well being may protect us from succumbing to illness or may lessen the severity if it occurs. Everyone knows that illness often comes after a period of unhappiness or stress. But that "from out of the mind", cited as a primary cause of MCS, or that our symptoms are purely imaginary do not hold water for me. I am convinced that physical illness does not arise from within the mind alone. But I will accept that emotional stresses may combine with internal and external physical factors to swing the balance towards disease.

In MCS external factors are the overwhelming

cause. When I suffered from migraines, a stressful happening such as abereavement or the threat of homelessness would be followed by an attack. However, once I had discovered and succeeded in avoiding the incitants, I found that even occurrences such as witnessing my husband's apparently lifeless body being removed from a North African swimming pool were no longer followed soon after or at all by migraine. When my body was no longer constantly struggling to resist an attack, the stress and shock no longer pushed it over into one.

No doubt some may say that a potent external factor could be suggestion; once the sufferer has heard of the condition they then develop the symptoms. But the patient needs to have heard of the condition first. It's unlikely that we all had. I certainly did not until I was diagnosed. Do people who are happily and successfully living their lives suddenly retreat into a restrictive illness that provides them with no sympathy or other benefit?

My symptoms were far worse when I knew nothing of the condition. Now I understand it to some degree, I am able to ameliorate some of those symptoms and am able to set out to advise and, I hope, help others. There would certainly be no gain in imagining or spuriously professing to have the condition: only loss. It has been described as just that; loss, loss, loss. I cannot believe that anyone not suffering the genuine effects from chemical exposures would tolerate the lifestyle and sometimes near opprobrium that results.

I was interested to note, when I began to talk to others who might be said by some only to "claim that they are suffering from MCS", that although we are all different, nevertheless I was hearing, at base, the same story of exposure followed by major problems time and time again. Some had been in contact with one another but only after the problems had arisen. I thought, "If I were a sceptic I would believe the condition was real now." It is easy to be sceptical about something that does not happen to match ones preconceptions. It may seem unacceptable. The proliferation of MCS is far from pleasing. We already have an allergy epidemic. Is the thought, that added to this more and more people are disabled and isolated by encountering common chemicals such as those from body care products, motor vehicles, household cleaners et al, that are such a feature of contemporary life, a comfortable one? It would be more comfortable to deny it.

I sincerely hope that although some MCS patients suffer from psychiatric symptoms this will not blind any physicians to the physical origins and physiological reality of these and other symptoms they may suffer. Perhaps it will be useful for me to append the following list. These are conditions to which in earlier days a psychogenic cause was originally attributed. Psychogenic, although strictly should not mean that the illness does not exist, has a connotation that it might not and somehow if the sufferers "got their acts together" and "got on their bikes", they would not be ill.

1. Multiple sclerosis
2. Parkinson's disease
3. Lupus
4. Interstitial cystitis
5. Migraine
6. Rheumatoid arthritis
7. Asthma
8. Gastric and duodenal ulcers
9. Ulcerative colitis

*PERSONAL VIEW* – *With women in mind,* Milica Brozovic, *British Medical Journal,* Volume 299, (9 September 1989)

# HAS THE ANSWER TO ALL THIS BEEN FOUND?

Dr Martin Pall, Professor Emeritus of Biochemistry and Basic Medical Science of Washington State University, has found that short term stressors that cause multisystem illnesses like MCS act by raising nitric oxide and peroxynitrite levels in the body. Following this a vicious cycle of mechanisms cause this to continue resulting in chronic illness. He has linked this to Chronic Fatigue Syndrome, MCS, Fibromyalgia, Post-traumatic Stress Disorder, Gulf War Syndrome and others. If this is at last concrete proof of MCS being of physiological origin this is a great step forward;

amelioration, even cure, may follow. But, meanwhile, we all will have to continue living with the condition.

*Explaining "Unexplained Illnesses"*
*Disease paradigm for Chronic Fatigue Syndrome, Multiple Chemical Sensitivity, Fibromyalgia, Post-traumatic Stress Disorder, Gulf War Syndrome and others.*
Martin Pall PhD, Professor Emeritus of Biochemistry & Basic Medical Science, Washington State University, USA.

## SUMMARY DEFINITION OF MCS

The symptoms occur in the presence of chemical exposure but in the absence of those incitants the symptoms resolve. Some find they are less affected by exposure when in a purer atmosphere. There is some suspicion that other unknown toxins may be involved. It is known that some atmospheric pollutants combine to produce others.

Symptoms occur at lower levels of exposure than previously tolerated by that individual.

Symptoms occur in response to a number of chemically unrelated substances and they involve multiple organ systems.

It is a chronic condition.

The symptoms vary from one individual to another but can be expected to remain the same for one individual for most of the time although it is also possible that a switch to other symptoms can occur.

As far as I know no research is being conducted in the UK. Most available information seems to originate in the USA.

There is a likelihood of some involvement of the central nervous system in the production of symptoms following chemical exposure.

## EXAMPLES OF THE SYMPTOMS

No individual will suffer them all.

- Breathing difficulties – blocked nose, various ear, nose and throat symptoms, asthma and other chest condition
- Skin rashes, inflammation of skin or mucosa
- Headaches, often severe
- Nausea, vomiting, bloating and other digestive problems
- Extreme fatigue, weakness, exhaustion, lethargy, inability to remain awake
- Insomnia
- Light headedness, fainting
- Joint and other pains
- Depression, anxiety, irritability, psychiatric symptoms
- Difficulty in concentration and the brain fog. This occurring in children will inhibit learning

- Influeza like symptoms
- Anaphylaxis.

One study reported that 77% of MCS sufferers had central nervous system problems, 45% had respiratory symptoms and 44% had gastro-intestinal symptoms.

If exposure to incitants is frequent or constant then fatigue, lethargy and malaise may be continuous.

## THE RESULTS OF MCS

Apart from the actual illness, those suffering it also suffer results from it. They may be too ill to work or may have to take lower paid or part time employment to accommodate their needs. Problems of travel isolate them from their friends and relatives. The latter may not understand the condition and consider them obsessive, reject them or harass them. Living with someone with the condition is difficult and complicated particularly when there is also a family growing up in the home. Accessing medical treatment, because of travel problems and problems of pollution in the buildings in which it is available, can seem formidable. Additionally, the fact that the condition may not be accepted as real is a major problem. Those with the condition must live in constant vigilance in order to avoid or cope with incitants.

# TREATMENT – PLUS SOME SUGGESTIONS

*(See also Coping wth the Condition)*

As yet there seems to be no cure. Identification of the main incitants and strategies for avoiding them and others although paramount are difficult. Actual scientific proof is hard to come by as there are so many variables in the environment. If the air quality was pure enough to obviate extraneous gases it is likely that any reaction would be muted. Most of us manage to discover the incitants by circumstantial evidence. Challenges to our assumption inevitably occur and prove them mostly all too correct.

We rely heavily on the cooperation of others around us. Confirmation of the diagnosis and advice from a physician specialising in the diagnosis and treatment of allergies is highly valuable. Advice over individual problems and some symptomatic treatment from an understanding General Practitioner is the greatest boon. Often traumatised in their past experience by disbelieving health professionals, it is difficult to overemphasise the value of these last two to MCS victims. Unfortunately not all of us have been diagnosed by a physician who understands the condition. I am one of the lucky ones and he was able to give me some useful advice. The consultation, although it did not result in a cure, was a healing experience.

Patients may have vitamin deficiencies, especially of

the B group, so dietary supplements may be of use. A course of vitamin $B_{12}$ by intramuscular injection is suggested by some writers. It is possible that a course of pantothenate acid (vitamin $B_5$) may aid general well-being.

Magnesium may help. This is based on the theory that MCS may be caused by elevated nitric oxide levels in the body and that magnesium would lower them (See above "Has the answer to all this been found?"). Some writers say that westerners are deficient in magnesium. Magnesium compounds can be laxative and by causing food to pass more quickly through the intestines have been accused of causing food allergies. However, eating magnesium rich foods such as figs, lemons, grapefruits, apples, nuts and seeds, and dark green vegetables may be useful.

Some sufferers claim that desensitisation has helped. But this may be risky.

Antihistamines can also be useful on some occasions although this has been disputed.

At the time of writing, based on the apparent neurological factor, a trial using a transcranial pulsed electromagnetic field is proposed in Denmark. This is similar to but a lighter form of treatment than the Electro Convulsive Therapy used to treat depression. Time will tell if this is efficacious. At present it tells us that in Denmark the condition is taken seriously.

*Transcranial pulsed electromagnetic field for Multiple Chemical Sensitivity; study protocol for a randomised double blind, placebo controlled trial* – Marie Thi Dao tran, Sine Skovbjerg, Lars

Arendt-Nielsen, Jasper Elberling. Trials – online journal Vol.14. 7th Space Interactive – press release.

More needs to be known about the condition.

# THE ROLE OF HEALTH PROFESSIONALS

As someone once said, being told that they need to be admitted to hospital will cause anxiety to anyone but to the MCS sufferer such words are a knell of doom. Not only will they be taken to a hostile environment full of hazards that can cause them unpleasant and even dangerous symptoms but they will be at the mercy of people who most likely will have no understanding of their condition. They may not even take it seriously making everything worse than it needed to be.

It is essential that everyone, even ancillary staff who may have only cursory contact with the patient or may have no direct contact but may enter their environment, understands the need for protection from incitants at all times. At the outset a nurse should have a thorough discussion with the patient or the person who knows them best and design a protocol for their care which must be communicated to all who will enter their environment.

Writing this of course is not enough. It must be strictly implemented. The importance of this must be made clear and suitable explanations given to those who, because of language or other impediment, may not understand written directives. A separate room with appropriate labelling is essential.

I spent twenty-four hours on an open ward. It is impossible to wear a vapour mask all the time because they restrict breathing and become too hot in the warm environment. I, therefore, had to keep a constant watch to be prepared to replace it when necessary. This became tiring and I could not have managed it if I had been really ill or if I had incitant levels there causing a need to wear a mask all the time. Some MCS sufferers are not able to tolerate masks and also, as we have to provide our own and they are expensive, a period of days reliant on them could be financially prohibitive to some. Fortunately the staff were kind and the ward not unduly polluted. But I was unable to approach near even the closed door of the toilet because of the strong fumes of the air freshener issuing from it.

I have already described the worth to the patient of a believing, understanding General Practitioner. All health service personnel of all ranks who are training to treat or care for patients should be taught about MCS. Those already in post should take steps to understand it as it is a condition that may present in any specialty.

We know that at present there is no cure but we do ask to be protected from unnecessary danger and harm or seeming unkindness due to ignorance.

*Website: <mcs-america.org/MCSHospitalPatientProtocol.Pdf>*

# CHEMICALS IN THE ENVIRONMENT – PAST AND PRESENT

*"Civilisation makes you sick"*
*Paul Gaugin*

As a victim it is easy to rail against chemicals but one must acknowledge their important uses and our dependence upon them in modern life. However, they have a negative side.

## SOME CHEMICAL SUBSTANCES COMMONLY AT FAULT IN MCS

Antiseptics, disinfectants, vehicle exhausts, perfumes and vapours from body care products, paints, herbicides, pesticides, household cleaning products, solvents and wood preservers are all commonly complained of by MCS sufferers. As there are so many chemicals in everyday use at present and most of the increase happened in the second half of the last century, there has not been enough time for their long term effects to be learnt. Heat causes more vapours to be given off. So a person or object that seems to be free from them may start giving off incitants when they become hot. Examples are after someone has taken exercise or when something is placed on a radiator.

## FORMALDEHYDE

It is a pungent odorous gas and is produced in vast quantities commercially to be used to make numerous chemical compounds which are used widely in manufacturing. Some examples of their use are resins and plastics, finishes to make fabrics crease resistant and components for motor cars. It is also used in photography. Its disinfectant quality results in the inclusion of its derivatives in many cosmetic and personal hygiene products to prevent growth of harmful bacteria. It is also used as a biocide to kill bacteria for the production of vaccines and to kill any contaminants that might occur. Mixed with water as formalin it was used to preserve biological specimens.

Highly volatile, it easily vaporises into the atmosphere from any substance that includes it and has become a common indoor pollutant. Formaldehyde has been blamed for childhood asthma and is suspected of being carcinogenic although as far as I know the evidence for the latter, so far, is not very strong. It is no longer allowed in Medium-Density Fibreboard, usually known as MDF, which is used in furniture, for example in fitted bedrooms and kitchens. It was found to cause nasal problems when used in the construction of mobile homes in America.

Formaldehyde is also present in cigarette smoke and may enter the atmosphere as a breakdown product of some substances such domestic cleaning agents. Urea-formaldehyde foam insulation was at one time pumped into cavity walls of houses to prevent heat loss. Initially it would give off formaldehyde and cause problems but once it set it became inert. However, should it become damp, formaldehyde is once more released into the atmosphere.

## BRONOPOL

This is a highly active antimicrobial compound so is therefore very useful as a preservative in cosmetics and shampoos and also some disinfectants and household cleaning agents. However, as it decomposes it liberates low levels of formaldehyde. Unfortunately low levels are too high for some of us.

## METHANOL

Widely used in chemical manufacture, can change into formaldehyde in some situations.

# AIR FRESHENERS

The first point about these is that they do not freshen the air at all. They are heavy pollutants masking the smell of stale air and other pollutants. They are supposed to be used in well-ventilated areas but usually in my experience they are used instead of ventilation in tiny toilet cubicles and other enclosed areas.

They seem to be of three types; hand-operated sprays, static containers giving off vapours constantly and those which are plugged into an electricity socket and pump out fumes periodically. Highly sensitive to them all, they are the bane of my life. I could find ways of coping with most incitants but the overuse of these items in almost all public toilets makes it difficult to go out and about. Often even my most powerful mask is not enough protection.

Hospitals are major culprits in this. The use of air fresheners in both public and private institutions seems to be completely unplanned and unregulated and appears to be the decision of the cleaners. Often these people are unaware of how heavily they are using them. I am told that often they spray them excessively as they leave an area, quite unaware of the overpowering result, waste of chemicals and that they are preventing a section of the population from using the facility they have cleaned.

I have even, on occasions, had to leave my local hospital whilst an outpatient, to look for a toilet to use elsewhere; once walking to the house of a kind friend and another time having my need accommodated, after some searching, at a church hall that happened to be open at the time. I have now found that their use in the building varies from department to department and recently, with some searching and advice from the staff, I have found a facility that I can use. Toilets apart, many people see fit to install or spray air fresheners randomly and unexpectedly. So a building that seemed safe to visit one week may not be the next. Also vice versa; so sadly one may avoid it unnecessarily.

One woman, to whom I spoke, fortunately not badly affected by chemicals on the whole, nevertheless had problems with the air fresheners about in the hospital where she worked. But fortunately, as a money saving exercise, they discontinued their use to her gratitude and benefit. A similar occurrence happened at my bank. The manager averred that it was necessary for the good of his customers to have one in the main public area but after a few months it disappeared and has never been replaced.

A study of children in Bristol linked air fresheners to diarrhoea and earache in children and headaches in their mothers. Naphthalene phenol, creosol, dichlorobenzene, xylene plus perfumes are found in them making them a toxic mix. If pinene and lemonene are ingredients, they easily react with any ozone present to create formaldhyde.

*Bristol children of the 90s' study,* Dr Alex Farrow, Archives of Envionmental Health (October 2004), reported by Nigel Hawkes in *The Times* (19 October 2004)

## PERFUMES

Perfumes, once, for most, a rare luxury, are now ubiquitous in our environment. There has been an explosion of artificially produced perfumes which are not only pervasive and long lasting but spread and remain widely throughout the area in which they are used. Many people complain of the discomforts they cause. Those with MCS can suffer real illness even to anaphylaxis. They may, of course, also be intolerant of natural perfumes because of their allergenic nature and the apparent tendency of those with MCS to develop more sensitivities as they go along.

Although the perfume wearers themselves appear unaffected it appears that they do absorb chemicals from these products. There are a vast number of perfumes and, although that word or the French "parfum" may occur in the ingredients listed on a wrapper of a preparation, the actual one is likely not to be identified. In 2012 an advisory committee of the European Commission advised restriction on some ingredients of perfumes. It is expected that new regulations will be proposed in 2014.

*The Times* (6 November 2012). See also – *The Growing Problem with Fragrance,* Alex Gazzola, *Journal of Action Against Allergy No 107,* (spring 2013), and – *Our Fetish for Fake Smells,* Ziauddin Sardar, *New Statesman* (1996) Vol. 129, issue 4503, makes interesting reading.

# DIVERSION INTO THE PAST OR HONEYMOONS THAT WENT WRONG

The use of chemicals increased as Western society became more industrialised and chemicals became cheaper and more readily available. Life changed, people could have and do things that had never been possible before. Now our lives are heavily dependent on chemicals and the products they have made possible by their use. Figures vary but it has been estimated that since the Second World War some 70,000 new chemical compounds have been developed. Many of these have found their way into products we use in our homes. But what is it doing to us and our environment? I am now diverting to look at some of them.

## LEAD

Industrial diseases due to exposure to some substances may date back to when humans discovered how to manufacture items from substances other than stone and wood. Lead, being a soft, malleable metal, came early into use by mankind. But once it is absorbed it accumulates in the tissues. It is poisonous and can damage the nervous system and cause blood disorders. Lead poisoning as such is most unpleasant and can be fatal when high enough levels are ingested. I wondered about the kohl, which the ancient Egyptians put around their eyes to protect them from the sun and disease, which contained lead. However, a well known Egyptologist has told me that it is likely that, as life expectancy was so short for them, the wearers and also the producers would have died from other reasons before chronic lead poisoning occurred. Lead vessels used for wine have in the past been cited as causal in the fall of the Roman Empire although this seems not to be considered to be an important factor now.

Potters used to suffer from a condition known as Lung Rot due to lead vapour from the glaze. Water pipes in houses were made of lead in the nineteenth and twentieth centuries. Lead could leach into the water, particularly in soft water areas. Children chewing items such as the bars of their cots were poisoned by the lead in the paint. This stopped when it became the norm to use lead free paint for anything with which children might come into contact and there was a phasing out of lead water pipes.

Lead was added to all petrol for many years resulting in lead pollution of the environment especially in urban areas. Children absorb higher levels of lead than adults and it impairs their learning ability and impulse control. By 1982, it was being said that nearly all urban populations had pathologically high levels of lead in their bodies; women being more sensitive to it but men accumulating more. After much campaigning, lead free petrol finally became available.

# MERCURY

*(see also MODERN TOXIC SOUP)*

Hat makers who were using mercury often became mentally ill: hence the term "mad as a hatter". It is now thought that King George the Third (Mad King George) was suffering from a condition known as "porphyria" which ran in his family. However, the fact that it began so late in life has led to speculation that, although he would have carried the appropriate gene, the condition might not have developed had he not ingested mercury through his scalp from the powder which was being applied to his wigs. A past method for clearing bedbugs from the bedstead was to mix quicksilver, as mercury was known, with the white of egg and apply it to all the cracks. Hopefully this damaged only the bedbugs. The Victorians used a mixture of mercury and chalk as a purgative for children, even royal ones.

*Queen Victoria's Youngest Son* by Charlotte Zeepvat, (Sutton Publishing, 1998), ISBN 0 7509 3791 2

# ARSENIC

Napoleon Bonaparte, at death, was found to have high levels of arsenic in his body leading to a suspicion that he had been poisoned. However by his time arsenic had become easily available and was commonly used in manufacturing processes. It was used in green dyes. There were reports of deaths due to exposure to the arsenic from those which were even used in clothing fabric. It was also used to produce green wallpaper. Even William Morris dyes had arsenic in them. The wallpaper could emit a poisonous vapour leading to chronic poisoning. Some Victorians, lying ill in their bedrooms, were unaware that the very paper that beautified their walls and even the paint on the window frames were the causes of their mysterious maladies. Arsenic would have been present in the dust that conscientious housewives wiped from ledges and with so much of it in the atmosphere it must have inevitably even fallen into food at times.

Arsenic, in its heyday, was also used in medicines. Charles Darwin's ill health, in the years subsequent to his famous expedition on the Beagle, may have been due to the arsenic which was used to treat his eczema whilst at university. It was easily acquired and used as a poison by Victorian murderers. As the symptoms of arsenic poisoning are similar to cholera, a disease familiar to all Victorian physicians, foul play might well not be suspected. Also there were many reported cases of accidental poisoning, as in the days before universal literacy it was mistaken for salt, sugar and even flour. Arsenic is still used today – in wooden garden dividers.

Christopher Catling – *Current Archaeology* Issue 243, (June 2010)

# AIR POLLUTION

*(see also MODERN TOXIC SOUP)*

As cities and towns grew, their inhabitants became more and more reliant on burning coal for heating and cooking. As early as 1306 Edward I briefly banned coal fires in London and Queen Elizabeth I banned burning coal in London when Parliament was sitting. By Victorian times "pea soup" fogs, when the air was laden with high humidity combined with smoke and fumes, were common in the capital and other large urban areas. Visibility was so limited that bus conductors had to walk in front of the vehicle to guide the driver. Experiences such as my mother's in the 1920s, when she thought she had become completely lost only to find that she was, in fact, standing beside the railings of the very house where she lived, were common.

Later, a government initiative to boost the coal industry by encouraging people to burn cheap coal resulted in the Great London Smog of 1962 which is famous for causing the deaths of about 4,000 people in four days and some 8,000 from its effects in the ensuing weeks and months. The Clean Air Act had already been passed in 1956 introducing smokeless zones and a thick, visible fog like that has never been witnessed in the capital since. But there was already a high level of pollution by vehicles' emissions and that has continued to increase since. This is not visible. But, some good news; Spheroidal Carbonaceous Particles

(SCPs) are produced by high temperature burning of fossil fuels and their presence in the atmosphere indicates air pollution. A study at the Lochnagar Basin in the Cairngorms showed an increase of them had occurred rapidly in the nineteenth century but there had been a fall around 1980 due to the Clean Air Act. Nevertheless in April 2014, *The Times* related that air pollution was killing 29,000 Britons each year.

*Tales from the Swamp* by Sebastian Payne, *British Archaeology*, (July/August 2005)

## ASBESTOS

At one time asbestos was considered the best thing *before* sliced bread. This naturally occurring mineral is resistant to heat, electricity and sound, making it very useful for insulation plus other uses such as in brake linings. Most people of my age will remember seeing asbestos, often crumbling, on domestic ironing boards. However, most roses have thorns and it became apparent that inhaling perhaps only a small amount of the fibres could cause mesothelioma and those working with asbestos often sustained this or other forms of lung malignancy or lung damage. Now there is strict legislation regarding asbestos and although present in many buildings, if it remains undamaged, usually with a protective covering, it is safe.

# THE MODERN TOXIC SOUP

We are said to live and learn, but do we? The above are some of the mistakes our forefathers made. But we are not any cleverer today which is sad seeing the vast progress there has been in scientific knowledge. There have been similar honeymoons with other substances or products. Examples from recent times are the original form of cling film which turned out to be a danger to health and the assurances given to the inhabitants of Camelford in 1988, when aluminium sulphate was accidentally added to their water supply.

Awareness of the pollution caused by motor vehicles has been a cause of anxiety for some decades. I, myself, supported the movement to get lead out of petrol when we discovered the high level of lead in the playground of the infant school which our children attended. But vehicle emissions still contain ozone, oxides of nitrogen, sulphur dioxide, carbon monoxide and hydrocarbons, all of which menace the health and well-being of those who inhale them regularly.

There is particular concern in London at present over the high levels of PM10 particulates breaching the European Commission's air quality standard. Air pollution in the streets is said to cause the deaths of 4,000 Londoners annually from lung cancer and asthma related conditions. This is mostly due to vehicle emissions. Diesel engines release vastly more carbon particles than petrol powered engines and are blamed for allergic reactions such as asthma.

A team of researchers reported to *The Lancet* online in January 2007 that Californian children who lived within 555 metres of motorways had significantly lower lung volume and peak flow than those who lived more than 1,500 metres away. When this was reported in *The Times* a spokesman for Asthma UK was quoted as saying that 66% of asthma sufferers reported that traffic fumes made their symptoms worse. In a study of air pollution and cognitive function Dr Jennifer Ailshire at the University of Southern California is reported to have found that increased exposure to air pollution decreases cognitive function in people aged fifty and over. A rise in air particle exposure of 10 micrograms per cubic metre was linked to a drop in cognitive function equivalent to ageing nearly three years.

Modern smog is described as photochemical smog. It results from sunlight hitting various atmospheric pollutants forming a mix of harmful chemicals. Fumes from industrial processes may add to this. Photochemical smog is an irritant to the air passages, causing disease and is also said to trigger heart attacks. Various strategies are to be employed to lessen this, such as spraying calcium powder on the streets to stop particles circulating in the air, planting more trees and creating more traffic free areas.

Hay fever, as it became to be known, was first described 200 years ago. But then there were very few cases although, interestingly, those described were from an urban population. Now it is said that one quarter of the UK population suffers from it and modern research has shown that there are higher levels of it in cities. As it is possible for traffic pollution to trigger plants to produce pollen with more allergic chemicals, it is postulated that pollution could be making humans more sensitive to pollen.

*Weather Eye*, Paul Simons, *The Times,* (2 July 2012)

## MODERN POLLUTANTS WHICH CAN CAUSE PROBLEMS

### OZONE

Some of us grew up believing that this was something beneficial to us to be breathed in at the seaside. But that which one smells at the seaside is likely to be rotting seaweed. Ozone is odourless but poisonous causing problems for those with breathing difficulties and it is thought to damage rubber, nylon, plastic, dyes and paint. It can be found in small quantities everywhere but is concentrated in the stratosphere fourteen miles above the earth where it forms a barrier against ultra violet radiation. But sea salt, ships' fumes and city smoke can lead to a chemical reaction that facilitates the formation of ozone smog at ground level. So ozone pollution is likely to be worse near ports.

Photocopiers, laser printers and high voltage electrical equipment can also produce ozone which is said to increase sensitivity to allergens. Ozone toleration varies between individuals but high levels can cause death. It is said to cause impaired lung function and cancer. Milder and more transient symptoms include coughing and wheezing and other breathing problems, headaches, dizziness, nausea, vomiting and inability to concentrate. It can also react with other pollutants. Older people are said to be more susceptible to ozone, which is said to be more toxic than chlorine, than younger people. The American Lung Association says there is no safe level for those with compromised immune systems.

## FORMALDEHYDE

Everyone knows this is a strong irritant and may have seen specimens preserved in it in a laboratory or museum. What is not known is that it is ubiquitous in our environment, particularly indoors. (*See CHEMICAL SUBSTANCES COMMONLY AT FAULT.*)

## INSECTICIDES

At present there is some concern over the falling numbers of honey bees. Seeds are often coated in insecticides which permeate throughout the plants. The neonicotinoids in the insecticides cause bees to forget where their food is. As bees are major pollinators this is a major problem for agriculturists. This is just one example of how the chemicals we use damage the environment.

## PESTICIDES

These might be suppressing our vitamin D levels. A Royal Society of Chemistry publication on the internet showed that adults with a high serum concentration of organ chlorine pesticides such as DDT also had lower vitamin D levels. In 2006 a team from Harvard School of Public Health was reported to have found a link with pesticides to the development of Parkinson's disease. They have a mixed bad and good press: bad for their possible bad health effects mainly to agricultural workers handling them or those living in proximity to fields; but good for improving produce yields. Those likely to be poor at detoxification will be wise to avoid them.

Study shows Parkinson's disease link to pesticides, Nigel Hawkes, *The Times* (26 June 2006)

# MERCURY NOW

Mercury as an alloy with another metal has been widely used for dental fillings. Some countries have discontinued its use but its likelihood of damaging the health of the individual, into whose teeth this silver-coloured substance, usually called dental amalgam, has been installed, is disputed. It is known that it is an environmental pollutant causing emissions of mercury during production and also during the cremation of corpses. This latter will be overcome as more crematoria install the appropriate equipment to trap it. Personally, I cannot believe that amalgam has been innocent; in my case, I passed my middle years with teeth heavily loaded with it and my better health now could be, at least in part, due to how few affected teeth I have left. It is accepted to sometimes have a battery-like effect when two teeth meet, causing migraines. As dentists are not in agreement about the safety of this compound it is best avoided.

# VOLATILE ORGANIC COMPOUNDS

These are carbon-based chemical compounds which have significant vapour pressure and thus can affect the environment and human health because they easily go into gaseous or vapour form, thus polluting the atmosphere. They are many, varied and everywhere, both man-made and naturally occurring. Indoors their concentrations can be highest although typically they are not acutely toxic. But exposure at low levels can produce chronic effects which develop slowly. Naturally occurring VOCs, as they are known, mostly come from plants: for example terpenes from which the paint thinner turpentine is made. Man-made VOCs include solvents, especially those used in paints and protective coatings and also chlorofluocarbons and halocarbons used in cleaning products and refrigerators. They are present in air fresheners, wood preservers, aerosol sprays, permanent markers, photographic solutions and can be given off when products are stored.

Commonly known VOCs are acetone, benzene, ethylene glycol used in antifreeze, formaldehyde (see above) and methylene chloride used in industrial processes. The term "Sick Building Syndrome" is well known. New furnishings, wall coverings and photocopiers can all give off VOCs. The level indoors can be up to five times higher than outside, sometimes even greater, and new buildings especially will have high levels due to the outgassing of their new components. In the home VOC levels are linked to the use of aerosols, air fresheners and carpet cleaner. VOCs are present in vehicle exhausts and cigarette smoke and can react with other gases to produce secondary ones. Some combine with nitrogen oxide to form ground-level ozone especially on hot sunny days.

VOCs can affect human health causing eye, nose and throat irritation; headaches; loss of coordination;

damage to the central nervous system, liver and kidneys. Also they can be responsible for skin reactions, breathlessness, nausea, vomiting, nosebleeds, tiredness and dizziness as well as affecting memory. These will all sound familiar to those with MCS. There is some proof that they can cause cancer in animals and they are suspected of doing similar in humans.

*Wikipedia: The United States Environmental Protection Agency*

## POLYCHLORINATED BIPHENYLS (PCBs)

These are compounds used in transformers, capacitors and coolants. They were used as plasticisers in paints and cements, casting agents, fire retardants, adhesives, waterproofing and railway sleepers. They share a structural similarity and toxic mode with dioxin. They were banned from use by the US Congress and the Stockholm Convention on Persistent Organic Pollutants in 2001. The UK had closed their use in new equipment in 1981 but use in existing equipment containing in excess of 5 titres PCBs was not stopped here until the end of 2000. I understand that their toxicity was known before their first commercial production but a conclusion was made that this was negligible. They affect the hormones in the body affecting development and can aid or cause malignancy to develop. Altered oestrogen levels can cause the feminisation of male foetuses or cause both sets of reproductive organs to develop. PCBs have been cited as causing damage to the nervous system as well. Although we can now hope that they are no longer used they still exist in the environment from their release during the time of their use and their later disposal.

*Wikipedia*

## PHTHALATES

These are mainly used as plasticisers; that is they are substances used to make plastics more flexible, long lasting and sometimes transparent. Primarily they are used to soften polyvinyl chloride (PVC). Health concerns have resulted in them being phased out of a number of products in the USA and the European Union but they will remain with us for some time. Some, from a long list of items in which they may be contained, are the enteric coating of pharmaceutical pills; adhesives and glues; building materials; medical devices for example catheters; detergents and surfactants packaging; children's toys; paints; printing inks and coatings; shower curtains; vinyl upholstery; floor tiles; food containers and wrappers, and cleaning materials. Many personal items such as perfume, eyeshadow, nail polish, hairspray and liquid soap are likely to contain them. They are also used in modern electronics. Phthalates are easily released into the environment. The good news is that they are easily broken down outdoors although concentrations of them in the external air are higher in populated areas. Because they are contained in so many everyday items it is not surprising that the amount of them in indoor air is generally higher then outside. They can easily leach and evaporate into food from PVC containers.

Most Americans who were tested by the Centers for Disease Control and Prevention showed signs of having absorbed phthalates. Although these are chemicals and are suspected of being harmful, possibly affecting hormone levels and even being responsible for the obesity epidemic, it seems that they are still mainly regarded as "suspects" but not yet proved guilty. It may also turn out that they are not involved with a precursor to Type 2 diabetes either as one study has suggested. However, it seems reasonable to advise those who have known sensitivity to chemicals that it is probably wise to avoid them as much as possible.

Polyethylene terephthalate ethylene (PETE) is used to make bottles for bottled water. There will be a "1" in the recycle triangle. Despite its name it should be free from phthalate plasticisers. PVC containers with a "3" in the triangle, I understand may leach phthalates.

*Wikipedia*

# SURFACTANTS

These substances are used in items such as detergents, fabric conditioners, paints, adhesives, ink, laxatives, some herbicides, insecticides, shampoos, conditioners, toothpastes and others. They can prove toxic to animals, ecosystems and, in sufficient quantities, to humans. Unfortunately, also, when in the environment, they can increase the spread of other contaminating substances.

*Wikipedia*

# DIOXINS

These are a well-known group of chemical compounds that persist in the environment as pollutants. They occur naturally. Examples of this are from forest fires and volcanic eruptions. Thus they have been with us at levels considered not to affect human health since the time of early man.

However, they result now from industrial activity too. At present 90% of human exposure to these highly toxic substances is through the food chain reaching us via meat and dairy products, fish and shellfish. Once absorbed they are said to have a half-life of seven to eleven years. Raised levels can cause reproductive and developmental problems, damage to the immune system, interference with hormones and also cancer. From time to time one reads in the press that human food has been contaminated by dioxins by routes such as the contamination of food fed to livestock.

*WHO Fact Statement N225* (May 2010 et al.)

## INDOOR POLLUTION

It is now accepted that indoors can be as much, indeed even more, polluted than outside. Partly I am sure it is because people do not ventilate their homes as once they did. This is due to unwillingness to lose heat both to save their pockets and, conscientiously, to lessen their carbon footprint. Sadly it is also true that we are all very much more now aware of security and the attraction that open windows have for unwanted intruders.

Our lifestyles and the consumer products now available seem to be the major culprits. We redecorate and refurnish more frequently these days using materials that give off vapours not previously encountered, especially when new. We use many more body-care products and these tend to be perfumed strongly with artificial perfumes and contain chemical preservatives. We use more and different chemicals in household cleaning. The so-called air fresheners are, as already mentioned, the bane of MCS victims' lives.

The demise of the open fire, welcomed by the housewife because of the dust and trouble it caused and by the environmentalist because of the pollution it caused, has also robbed the home of a useful ventilator. The heat drew stale air up the chimney and it is likely some gases were burned as they were sucked into the flames. Wind passing over the open chimney sucked air out of the house even at times when there was no fire. It worries me that children are exposed to far more chemicals now than we were, particularly as they are likely to ingest them more heavily than adults.

## ENDNOTE

As I am not scientifically qualified I have tried not to overstate the negative side of modern chemicals. Perhaps I have been too careful; perhaps not. They have caused a wonderful revolution in the way we live during the last seventy years but it is too soon for us to know the long-term effects. But with so many powerful substances introduced into the environment, outdoors as well as in, over a short time span, is it surprising that some of us are physiologically unable to cope? The West and increasingly the rest of the world have embraced the chemical revolution wholeheartedly where perhaps caution should have been paramount. Now we have discovered that some can cause cancer, others reduce fertility and have other hormonal effects with also perhaps even obesity... A number, which seems to be increasing, find they have a crippling sensitivity to chemicals. This does not mean that all chemicals are necessarily bad. Like dogs, which as a nation we love, wrongly or too excitedly handled they are likely to bite.

# THOSE AFFECTED SPEAK

I have omitted lists of symptoms and excitants from many of these accounts as they commonly equate to those already described. Some are from accounts written by the respondent, others have been written from notes I made during telephone conversations. I have written them as if the person was speaking but with great care as to factual accuracy. "M" indicates a man and "F", a woman is recounting experiences.

## F. 1

I had to retire early because the building where I worked made me ill. I cannot tolerate fire retardants, plastics, dyes, soap powder, some medicines, gas and electric heaters. Sodium lauryl sulphate is a problem. My reactions are asthma, repeated chest infections, eczema, swelling of the face, a feeling of being drained and a tendency to lose consciousness. The new central heating caused me to become unconscious. I need to wear goggles to shop and I have to line all my clothes with pure silk; also, to make my own bra because of the latex. I was diagnosed by a doctor. My GP is understanding, as was the first allergist, but my new allergist is not. I had to discontinue a degree course because of MCS and Electrical Sensitivity which I also suffer from. These also prevented my dentist from filling a tooth. He just had to file it off. I am also gluten and lactose intolerant. I live alone and am isolated by the condition. I cannot visit my children or go on holiday. My daughter understands but my son does not believe the condition exists.

## M. 1

I am elderly. I worked in the petroleum industry. I have had MCS for some time and now have other medical conditions. Food intolerance has become a major problem. My advice to others is "God loves a trier".

## F. 2

I developed MCS in 1998 after having ME since 1991. Then, I was still able to tolerate normal exposure to chemicals except cigarette smoke which immediately caused a tightening of the chest. Otherwise I could socialise freely. In 1998 I inadvertently inhaled smoke from a burning joss stick in an adjacent room at a friend's house. A sleepless night followed with a tight chest, shortness of breath and fearfulness. After a few days I visited my GP who told me I had mild asthma and prescribed inhalers. I persevered with these for thirteen awful days. My bronchial tubes felt as if they were full of sand, I suffered sleeplessness, nightmares and hallucinations, palpitations, headaches and overwhelming fear. During this time different asthma drugs were tried but nothing helped. So I stopped the inhalers and immediately these symptoms eased.

I cannot remember when I first heard the term MCS but it must have been whilst researching allergies. I observed my reactions to everything in my life – my home, my leisure pursuits and my outdoor activities. It became clear I had two distinct sets of reactions. One set of reactions was based on my breathing; tightness in my upper chest, a feeling that I could not breathe properly, a need for cool, fresh air and a production of white phlegm obstructing the airways and, after lying down overnight, an over-active sense of smell.

The second set of reactions involved headaches, light headedness, feelings of panic and loss of control, sleeplessness, fearfulness and tearfulness. These latter reactions seemed to be triggered by more volatile chemicals such as unburned petrol, perfume, new car smells and paint fumes.

MCS turned me into a fearful recluse. Wherever I was, I was on "red alert" for the slightest smell. The resultant stress did not improve my chronic fatigue condition. I could not go into anyone's car because of the gases from the glues and upholstery; I could not walk in the street because of the car fumes. Papers and magazines outgassed ink and paper smells. The smell of people's clothes, due to the perfumes in washing powder, is still the most unpleasant thing to deal with. However, I have managed over the years to sort out what I can do, and to do it well, and not moan over what I cannot do.

The first thing was to attend to my home environment. I use safe cleaning products and cook with a *Remoslea* – a lovely little pan and grill arrangement which cooks almost anything with almost no cooking smells. My fan oven which caused a lot of problems is never used. I banished pine furniture from my bedroom and when furniture and fittings have to be renewed I do a lot of research first. No one uses perfumes or aftershaves in my company – even people visiting to give quotations or do jobs in the house are politely asked not to wear them. Friends and family know to obey these simple rules. It was hard at first but I have to be strong, though I still cannot get my daughters to use "safe" washing powder.

I feel that, through excluding as many inhaled toxins as possible, over the years my tolerance has become stronger. I still experience the reactions I have described on a daily basis but the fear and panics have gone. I have come to terms with MCS. I have had it for twelve years and it hasn't killed me yet!

Regarding hospital experience, I had a mastectomy in 2005. The anaesthetist was perturbed about my possible reactions to the anaesthetic, but although I felt quite nauseated afterwards, I came through it. It is vital to discuss the problem with everyone concerned. I was able to have a private room with a large notice on the door, "Do not enter if wearing perfume". Chemotherapy and radiotherapy affected me but probably similarly to other people. But I could not tolerate the anti-sickness drugs. I would say to anyone with MCS, who is fearful of hospital treatment, share your fears, explain your difficulties; the hospital staff will do their utmost to accommodate you.

We purchased a second-hand caravan a few years ago and I use it as a bolt-hole when work is being done on the house. But even though we used special paint in the kitchen I was three months before I could safely use it. I would love to find "safe" holiday accommodation other than the caravan but have yet to find anywhere catering for someone with such extreme sensitivities. People advertising holiday accommodation on the allergy sufferers' website seem to consider a carpet-free bedroom to be the answer.

My encouragement to all MCS sufferers is to regard it as a challenge rather than as an affliction.

## F. 3

My doctor did not understand and thought that I had "fanciful ideas" and I won't talk to him about it again. A friend diagnosed the problem from a magazine article. Woodworm treatment in the house made me really ill. I had to give up my office job to work as a postwoman. My social life suffers and I have to wash new clothes six times and I can't always wear them then. I can go on holiday if I camp and there is one holiday cottage where they accommodate my needs. Fortunately my partner and children are very supportive.

# M. 2

Our trouble is that we look normal but I go into anaphylaxis. My wife has to come with me carrying an EpiPen if I go out. The carer is the one who suffers most. I am unconscious and so unaware of what is happening. One of my triggers is spices. Pepper on my food can send me to hospital. I am affected by numerous things including perfume.

When I have to go into hospital I need a separate room which my wife has to clean first as the materials they will use put me into shock. After work each day she needs to go home and cook special food for me as the hospital cannot guarantee to provide me with safe food. Staff do not look at my bracelet or even the information in my notes about MCS. I have had the condition for twenty years. I think it was caused by exposure to perfume and cigarette smoke at my workplace. I have become adjusted to my restricted lifestyle but it is sad not to attend one's children's weddings.

## F. 4

I cope with the chemical problem by avoidance but I have great difficulty with food although I can eat out, but with difficulty. Roasts suit me best but I must avoid sauces and spices. I only weigh five stone. Candida is a problem. I ask my carers not to wear perfume.

## F. 5

I am hypersensitive to chlorine, formaldehyde, paints, wood preserver, air fresheners and chemical perfumes. Towns are a problem; the diesel and petrochemical exhausts cause my eyes to stream and become inflamed. I am intolerant of a number of foods including chemical flavourings. Things in meat, from the animals' feed, cause abdominal pain. I have arthritis and IBS. I was a teacher but could not work full-time. By being peripatetic I could have fresh air between classes. My colleagues were supportive, understanding my particular needs over refreshments, for example as I am intolerant of tap water I provided my own. They warned me if paint or glues were being used. Even starting work late and only doing part-time, I was "washed up" by the end of the day. We have a caravan for our holidays and I can stay in hotels if the housekeepers vacuum the mattress first. I have problems with feather pillows and new mattresses. I suffer from low blood pressure. My husband is a "brick" and my doctor has been sympathetic.

## M. 3

The condition started in about 1991. It is difficult to be precise because I did not understand what was happening at the time. My symptoms occur in the following order as exposure increases:

- Tinnitus
- Prickly face around nose, mouth and cheeks
- Prolonged exposure causing my face to become red and feel sore
- Drowsiness
- Loss of energy
- Shivering
- Depression
- Bad temper
- Aggressive behaviour

The symptoms do not go away until the cause is removed. Severe exposure will require hours spent energetically in the open air to clear the condition. It took two or three years before I could identify the problem. Suspecting allergies I consulted books and consequently went to Keighley Allergy Hospital where the problem was diagnosed and I received helpful advice. This was reassuring. I was not going mad after all.

I then had to identify the substances that affected me and this is ongoing. The list at present is:

- Dust mites
- Fire retardants and other chemicals in furniture, carpets, beds, etc.
- Air fresheners
- Cleaning fluids and detergents
- Bleach and disinfectants
- Paints and varnishes
- Printing ink
- Polishes, solvents and glues
- Perfumes
- Chemicals in new clothes
- Building materials, insulation, polystyrene, etc.

In the early stages, when we did not realize what was happening, the problem affected my wife almost as much as me. She didn't know what to do for the best. We suspected all manner of things to be causing my discomfort. We eventually moved, hoping to resolve the problem, to an old house. It had an open fireplace giving good ventilation which we knew would be helpful.

The ongoing effects remain considerable affecting us both. Examples are:

- I cannot tolerate new mattresses, bedding, furniture and carpets; we have to buy second-hand or antique, or, alternatively, store new items for several years before use.
- My sensitivity to dust mites increases my wife's workload in washing bedding and general cleaning.
- Holidays are a problem as the cleaning regime of hotels usually means lots of chemicals. We have learned to use rented apartments or cottages giving us more control over the environment. Even then we take our own bedding and hope the mattress is not new.
- My wife cannot use perfumes and we keep soaps and shampoos etc. to an absolute minimum.
- We have outside storage for chemicals.
- Our entire lifestyle has had to change and we have spent several thousand pounds trying to cope with the problem.

## F. 6

It's a nightmare. It ruined a marriage of thirty years. I am housebound and have stopped having a life. I can't travel. I can't tolerate magazines, plastic, rubber, etc. Perfumes are dreadful. I had to change my doctor because of air fresheners at the surgery and now I consult him by phone but do not mention MCS. It came on after a field next to here was sprayed. I am on a learning curve that I do not like to be on but I try to keep a sense of humour. I do worry about the children that are exposed to so many chemicals these days.

## F. 7

Chemical problems are fewer than the food ones at present and I am on a rotation diet. But it is a minefield. I cannot wear cotton, only wool and silk. Air fresheners are a problem. It is an isolating condition but I plod along and hope for the best.

## F. 8

The condition seemed to be triggered by new timber in the house treated with a pyrethroid when my immune system was already weakened by ME. It is isolating. Socialising is very limited – no visits to the shops, theatre, concerts, etc., and no travel. I miss live culture. The worst aspect is isolation. I am retired but would not be able to work. My advice to fellow sufferers is to make contact with others by phone. Spend time with nature, walk in the country, garden, and feed and watch the birds. Keep a pet and do creative handicrafts. Above all remember you are not alone. We are all going through this together.

## F. 9

My MCS could have been caused by new furniture but I did notice that when the farmer sprayed the field next to us the foliage on a tree in our garden always died. When we have been to the supermarket I have to wash mine and my husband's clothes. If I visit my daughter we leave our coats in the car so as not to pick up chemical gases from her house. I could not stay at her house and if they come to us we have to air our furniture out of doors afterwards. I can read library books and second-hand ones. I have problems with pine trees and pine wood. We had to change the wood in our caravan and we bought a summer house but I cannot use it. I cannot visit the hairdresser or go into other people's houses. I can't go away except in our caravan that has its own toilet and shower. Some doctors understand the problem. Others do not. The allergist was very rude to me about it. Travelling to see him had been difficult for me. So it was disappointing.

## F. 10

Various things affect me – chemical vapours and foods.

Living in a house with gas heaters made me depressed and my marriage broke up. I had to move to a house without gas. I have had to take an outdoor job with no office. Friends do not understand and my closest friends are unsympathetic. People can't understand vapour problems. I do not mention it to my doctor. It is easiest to keep quiet; even my parents did not believe me. I have had to find out about things myself and things are better than they were.

## F. 11

I was a nurse for many years but I can't enter a hospital now.

## F. 12

I can only go out to the park at certain times. A visit to Marks and Spencer would seem like a holiday.

## F. 13

I don't tell my doctor in case it compromises his attitude to my other conditions.

# F. 14 SO THAT'S WHAT'S WRONG WITH ME!

*The personal account of the author*

In the 1940s the housing stock was still depleted from the war. Just before my tenth birthday, we moved into a converted stable. The rooms were light and airy but our landlord kept his car in what, I believe, may have once been the tack room at one end. There were as yet still few cars on the roads but some of them were venerably ancient. His car would certainly have dated from the early 1930s, if not late 1920s. It had a dicky seat. It was noisy and when he ran it into the garage a very strong smell permeated the whole of our cottage. The yard in front, in which I played, was mostly enclosed by buildings. Delivery vans came in and out adding to the pollution. Also a man used it at weekends to clean and tinker with his sports car, often running the engine whilst stationary. In short we were subjected to considerable vehicle pollution.

The last year in my junior school I remember as very happy. Having gained a place, I was very much looking forward to going to grammar school, the sun shone and all seemed to be extremely well in my world. But this was like a lull before the storm.

I enjoyed my new school and the new and interesting subjects we studied. But, having always had little contact with other children, I was a bit of an oddity at school, having conversation and ideas influenced more by middle-aged adults than my peers. Not surprisingly I was teased. I had no strategies for defending myself and unfortunately in our form was a girl who had brought a reputation up with her from the junior department as troublemaker.

She had a very able lieutenant and they and their clique tormented me. Of course, to defend themselves from similar onslaughts, others joined in. It seemed at the time that I had the whole form against me but looking back I believe that was not so. But my hair was pulled, my possessions constantly hidden and damaged. I was particularly sensitive about damage to my uniform because I knew the difficulty my mother experienced in providing it.

Rude comments and name-calling for some reason did not trouble me. But I could never relax at school because I never knew what onslaught would occur next and there was no place I could go to be safe. As I lay down to sleep at night I would still feel my hair being pulled and my behind being pricked by drawing pins as they had been during the day. Although I did not yet know the word I became very tense. School had become a daily ordeal and there was no escape except mercifully at weekends.

I was intent on getting myself educated and also believed that if I did not go to school my beloved father would be sent to prison. Parental advice was that I should not be upset by a bit of teasing and that it must be my own fault that I was not popular. However, there was no indication given on how to overcome the latter. I was trapped!

The prolonged period of stress led on to periods of what I was later told was termed "dissociation" and was linked to the migraines I had already begun to experience, as well as anxiety. It would strike suddenly and unexpectedly. One minute all was well; the next I felt that I was no longer in the scene that I was beholding. It was the feeling of not being anywhere in heaven or earth, of being nowhere but feeling absolutely terrified. At eleven years of age I described it as feeling faint, not having the linguistic skills for an alternative. This was fortunate as I might well have been mistakenly thought to be psychotic and treated accordingly.

Our family doctor was very kind and repeatedly endeavoured to diagnose the infirmity which I was unable, adequately, to describe. However, my frequent retreat to sickbay when these attacks occurred in school became noticed and the school doctor referred me to a child guidance clinic. For a number of years I attended sessions there with a Jungian psychotherapist.

The stress eased in the second year when I was with a number of different companions and the frequency of these attacks decreased. Our landlord later changed to a modern car but they never stopped until a few weeks after I had left home at seventeen and the Jungian lady had long since given me up as a hopeless case.

I now feel convinced that, although stress no doubt

played a part, vehicle exhaust was the major factor. Exposure to high levels in a busy city street can result in light-headedness and a feeling of panic even now. Whereas milling crowds and numerous vehicles, when the pollution is not trapped between high buildings, do not affect me. It has been observed that slow-moving traffic affects children who have asthma more than that moving quickly on a dual carriageway. Seemingly, then, slow-moving traffic emits higher levels of pollution.

The trips to the psychotherapist, although they ate in to my school time and never approached the real problem, were not completely wasted. My symptoms had resulted in my being chivvied at home and, at school, led to the belief that I had an inadequate personality. She helped me regain some self-esteem and, although lack of finance prevented me doing a university course, I gained enough confidence to embrace an alternative career with some success.

But I had lost my adolescent years because of fear. Dissociation, when it happened away from home especially in a strange place, was really terrifying. There were, at that time, stories of people losing their memories and then finding themselves in strange towns many miles away; the thought this might happen to me during one of these occurrences frightened me very much at twelve and took until my late teenage years to overcome. I never went anywhere other than the local village and surrounding lanes except when I was unable to avoid doing so. So I never did the usual things that young people usually do when they are growing up, living as much like a recluse as I could.

But once I had moved out from home and started training as a nurse, although the migraines continued, life was much better. I was able to manage them fairly well. With only three exceptions in fifteen years I was always able to keep going until I came off duty and then be recovered enough to go back to work the next morning. Two of those exceptions were when I was discovered vomiting in the sluice and sent off duty despite my protestations.

I gained confidence to lead a more normal life; although I noticed that I needed to spend more of my off-duty time resting than did my colleagues, I kept up. The next downturn perhaps has had a more serious and prolonged effect than seemed at the time. Having developed cellulitis as a result of an injury during a car crash I was prescribed my first antibiotic. An almost immediate result was candida infections. What a nuisance they have been and how much has gut dysbiosis contributed to my MCS?

Through my late twenties I seemed to acquire an increasing number of minor symptoms. Collectively they never seemed to equate to any illness that I had heard of. But, as during my adolescence I had been thoroughly brainwashed into believing I was one of "life's inadequates", although puzzled by them I somehow accepted that minor ill health was my lot. At the same time, I was acquiring more and more amalgam fillings in my teeth on an annual basis. Mercury amalgam I feel sure, as I have said, is not innocent in my case. Not having had a migraine for some teens of years I had a severe and uncharacteristic one on the morning after the dentist had carefully drilled out a large piece of amalgam from a tooth.

But things really went wrong when I got married and we moved into a newly decorated flat with nearly all new furniture. As well as the pre-existing orchestra of symptoms, came fatigue, overwhelming lethargy and more frequent headaches. Fortunately I was between jobs. I tried to drag myself back to normal activity but it seemed that every time I made plans or an appointment my headache would be too severe for me to go. I made and cancelled so many appointments with my dentist that I became too ashamed to make any more. It was during this period that I had my first major reaction with prostration and shaking.

My years of motherhood were difficult, characterised by frequent migraines and what I now suspect were reactions to chemicals when we bought new items or decorated parts of the house. I could not understand why I suffered from short-lived flu-like illnesses when no one around did. My husband was wonderful. It was not unusual for him to come home after a day's work to find me pacing the floor to keep awake with a migraine or migraine-like condition. He would then take over caring for the children whilst I staggered off to bed.

Nothing I tried helped and prescribed medicines seemed to make the attacks worse. I frequently castigated myself for not doing as well as other women in my place, most of who, although they had children, also went out to work. Fatigue and lethargy were a daily problem. Fortunately, we had already decided that if children came I would remain at home. One day it dawned on me how many days a year I was losing to illness. However, that did not make me feel any less inferior. Nothing seemed to help the migraines until one day a friend told me about *Migraleve*. It was not infallible in my case but it worked quite often. Life and "productivity" started to look up.

But a great step forward was discovering that migraines could be triggered by food. I gradually discovered most of the triggers for the attacks and by avoiding them entirely I discovered what it was like to feel well – for most of the time anyway. I felt cheated. Most people were like this nearly all the time! Noting the link with candida I have, from time to time, managed a spell on an anti- candida diet. Even a month or so seems to me to help a little but I must confess I have never managed the six months or more that is probably necessary.

With good dietary control, despite being in my menopausal years, things seemed good. I decided that I was too out of date to return to being a sister tutor. I had had my hearing badly damaged by a missed infection, probably because of the same sort of misunderstanding that had marred the birth of my first daughter and had endangered us both. I feel that on both occasions my complaining of symptoms, which I now know are due to chemicals but for which no physical signs were evident, discredited me in the eyes of my medical attendants.

Deafness would have been a barrier to clinical nursing so I looked elsewhere. I was able to impress my adolescent children by getting myself both retrained and re-employed in one year. I began teaching adult literacy. I loved the work. Being a part-timer I had just the right balance of domesticity and outside interest. My past work experience seemed to have led seamlessly to this and maturity stood me in good stead with young male prisoners when I occasionally deputised for the prison tutors. To most of these prisoners I must have seemed older that many of their grandmothers.

But roses have thorns. I was sensitive to the whiteboard markers which we used. Of course it took a while to work out what was happening but one day I was presented with incontrovertible evidence. My seniors were very understanding and provided me with a chalk-only room to teach in. It was a bit shabby but my students generously accepted it. So we carried on.

Twenty years later I stay fairly well by dint of avoiding incitants. Being retired, avoidance is easier. The items that make me ill are legion but similar to those complained of by others. I could not manage any semblance of normal life without a vapour mask always available in my pocket, even at home. The ubiquitous air fresheners are my greatest problem and I am particularly sensitive to aftershave. I can handle minor reactions but a major prostrating one is always possible.

As I care for my husband I have to be careful to remain on my feet. So life is restricted but, as evidenced above, I am not alone. But the unnecessary deafness compounds my problems. I can manage fairly well in one-to-one situations but in a group or at the occasional lectures that I still manage to attend I commonly find myself unable to hear what is being said even with a digital hearing aid. I find this worse to bear than MCS as its contribution to my social isolation is greater.

My symptoms range from light-headedness, nasal inflammation, headaches, indigestion and tiredness to a full prostrating reaction as had happened whilst teaching when I had inadvertently run hot water on to the dust from a blackboard rubber that had become contaminated with whiteboard marker ink. Having felt very unwell all day, that evening I collapsed on my bed shaking and, although all I wanted to do was to lie still, I could not. I tossed and turned uncontrollably, shaking, retching and occasionally vomiting, my head aching. My husband wanted to call a doctor but it was after-hours and I forbade him, feeling that it would likely be a stranger who did not know me and I felt unable to once more face the "psychological business" which had happened at a similar incident previously. I will admit that the sight of me tossing about on the bed and retching, apparently exaggeratedly, might well have appeared histrionic. As usual with a severe reaction, after a time I fell irresistibly into the deep sleep which some of us term "passing out". On that occasion I had managed to get through the working day but now it seems to overcome me more rapidly.

Like others, I find brain fog can be a problem, especially when I am experiencing a reaction away from home, as it causes difficulty over deciding how to cope with the situation. Calling a taxi to take me home might aggravate the problem as there are air fresheners in many of them. Fear of this limits excursions of any distance from the safety of home. A greater grief to me is that, were it not for MCS, during the last sixteen years I could have been usefully active as a volunteer in the community using the experience and the skills I had developed during both work and childrearing. But the greatest grief is that MCS is not universally acknowledged in this country for what it is.

# COPING WITH THE CONDITION

*Warning – proceed thoughtfully with caution*

One's first reaction to the following may be, "Oh, I can't do all that". Of course you can't and moreover some of the advice that follows may not be useful or even safe for you as an individual; although helpful, I hope, to others. I have been collecting advice for MCS sufferers for over a decade. Needless to say I have not been able to test it all myself.

Please take most items of my advice as possibly helpful suggestions and consider carefully before undertaking anything written here. Although I have thought carefully as to its general safety before I have written this, I can take no responsibility if anything goes wrong as, with our varying sensitivities, what is safe for one may be perilous for another. But, hopefully, much that follows may prove helpful. If you are unsure, you may have a health professional that can advise you. Otherwise, miss it out or approach it very carefully.

My sympathies lie with those who feel frustrated because they cannot follow some of the advice as they would wish because they lack the necessary facilities, energy or finance. This is an expensive condition but sadly those who suffer from it are likely not to be well off. For example, the condition may have robbed them of their livelihood. Conversely, if we were rich and lived on large country estates it is likely we would not have contracted it anyway.

# ADJUSTMENT

If this condition has come upon you suddenly it is a shock and you and those close to you need to take time to adjust. But do not spend money feverishly on hoped for cures or equipment that will prove useless. Do not dwell on those aspects of life and freedom which you have lost. Accept that times are now, not what they were. But do concentrate on what you can still have and do. Look for other avenues. There may even be interests that you have always wanted to follow but have never before had the time. Perhaps they are still possible. Keep as busy and active as you can. It will keep your mind off your minor symptoms. You may not be able to visit your friends but hopefully you can still telephone or write to them. Encourage them to keep in touch. Try to seem cheerful even if you are not; as my mother often quoted, "Laugh and the world laughs with you. Weep and you weep alone." Although advice can be useful, expect to manage your own condition. If someone else took over they would be more restrictive than you will be to yourself.

# MAKING A START – DETECTION OF INCITANTS, AVOIDANCE AND PROTECTION

Take stock of your situation and as soon as you have a period free from brain fog (I think for most brain fog is only occasional), and having read through all of this, make a plan.

There are four main principles to follow:

1. Identify and avoid the causes of your problem.
2. Lessen the load of other chemicals on your body. Below are a number of ways of doing this. Although you will always need to strenuously avoid the real excitants, if you follow a low exposure regime at home you can relax your guard sometimes, when it seems more convenient to do so, in respect of these lesser threats.
3. Despite the difficulties try to live as normal and active a life as you can.
4. Do all you can to remain healthy in other respects. You have enough problems as it is. I hope to cover this further on. But one particular piece of advice to start with; always wash your hands, not only before eating, but when you return from being out. Viruses and other micro-organisms can live on surfaces for longish periods so you may never have seen the person from whom you caught flu but who left the infection on a door handle which you later touched.

The flu epidemic of a few years ago never reached the levels that were predicted. I wonder if it was because there was an energetic campaign urging hand washing. When you are out, if you are unable to use the soap provided, carry a little of your own with you in a small plastic box. Remember infection can get into your body not only from your fingers to your mouth but via your nose and eyes also. So, when out and about, keep your hands from your face.

## THE ARTICULATE ADVOCATE

In some circumstances, for example if you are unexpectedly admitted to hospital, it is useful to have someone such as a relative or friend to come with you who is able to describe your needs and will, if necessary, plead on your behalf for them to be met.

## A MEDALLION

Make sure that you wear some form of medallion carrying the information that you are very sensitive to chemicals. Also carry a list of them in your bag or wallet to show health professionals.

## KNOWING YOUR ENEMIES

To start at the beginning; first, of course, you need to know your enemies or at least where they are. Having read the sections on chemicals and other sufferers' experiences you will probably be getting some idea where to look if you did not know already. Be prepared that it may take time and you may make mistakes. Sometimes the circumstances in which reactions occur are quite obvious. The actual cause may be less so. Obviously try to avoid any situations that you know will cause your symptoms; if this is not possible, try to protect yourself when there. Whilst in the long run it is useful to name an actual incitant the most important thing at first is to find out where they are and then to avoid them. Knowing their names is secondary but useful when you need to tell others about it, for example health professionals. So keep notes when you get a reaction. Where were you? What was happening? What could have been giving off vapours? Soon you may see coincidences that guide you.

## AVOIDANCE AND PROTECTION

Avoidance is the only sure way of dealing with MCS. But this is not always possible. However, you can lessen exposure, to some degree, to vapours you cannot avoid with vapour masks.

# VAPOUR MASKS

The Healthy House supplies a choice of these and they can also be obtained through stockists of protective clothing for workmen. Those from the latter can vary from the lightweight, giving only light protection, to helmets designed for really toxic atmospheres. I find that a comfortable lightweight mask protects me from normal background pollution but I need a thicker one, as from the Healthy House, in the presence of a disseminator or air fresheners or other chemicals which give off a lot of fumes.

Some air fresheners, sadly, overwhelm even a heavyweight mask. In shops, check that they understand that you require vapour masks or you may be served paper masks used for dust pollution. Myself, I could not function without one or other of these readily available in my pocket at all times, even my dressing gown. At home one can be taken by surprise by a chance caller or someone opening a parcel and even pollution blown on the breeze.

Do not feel too embarrassed to wear a mask. Your friends will soon get used to it when they understand why. It is probably best to explain why you are wearing a mask when you meet people for the first time. Coloured masks are preferable when encountering strangers. White masks often convey the wrong message. It may be thought that one is neurotically fearful of infection or that one is oneself infectious. Health professionals can become irritated by the sight of them (see OTHER PEOPLE) if they do not understand.

## OTHER PROTECTION

A small amount of Vaseline petroleum jelly smeared inside the nostrils can give a little protection, whilst a silk handkerchief held bunched over the nose may help protect you from ambient vapours over a short period. When passing someone or something emitting noxious vapours you may be fortunate enough to be able to hold your breath until you feel it is safe.

## CUTTING DOWN YOUR CHEMICAL BURDEN

Think "chemical" at all times and not only avoid those that you know you must but, even if it seems safe, ask yourself "Is this one really necessary?" and if you cannot avoid, cut its use to a minimum. Aim in the direction of a pure uncontaminated body in a pure uncontaminated environment. It is likely that if we could actually achieve a completely contaminant-free environment we would lose our ability to detoxify them if we did meet them. However, as this is unlikely to occur and whilst we breathe the air around us, we will still meet contaminants. Most of which follows is aimed at helping you to lessen your chemical burden.

## A SAFE HOME

Try to eliminate as many chemical substances from your home as you can. For general safety no chemical substances should be stored under the stairs, particularly paint or spirit which would constitute an extreme hazard in the case of fire. But they are all likely to be emitting vapours into the atmosphere where ever they are kept although the shaking and vibration under stairs would increase this.

First, look at all cleaning agents and other chemicals that you have and think if they are really necessary. Dispose of as many as you can. If possible those you keep should be stored in an outside shed or garage. Indoors they should be shut away in a cool place away from sources of heat and, of course, where children cannot reach them. Even if you think a chemical is safe for you use it in as small a quantity as you can for it to be effective. Take the precaution of wearing a mask and do it outdoors if possible. I always clean shoes like that. Better still, let someone else, if they are willing, do it for you. May I repeat, if any chemical is used by you or anyone on your behalf it should be used in the smallest amount needed to be effective.

Minimalism is a key word for your living space too. Try to keep things as simple and uncluttered as you can. The more items around, the more chance that they may give off vapours, the fewer, the easier the place is to clean and thus saves your energy.

Newsprint should be removed from living areas as soon as it has been read and stored in a cool place before recycling. Many people have a problem with printing ink.

Be prepared to outgas new items before you put them to use. Only introduce them after you have assured yourself that they are safe.

Remember that heat causes chemical vapours to be given off faster. So watch that your possessions stay away from sources of heat such as radiators or sunshine coming through windows.

So make a careful assessment of your home and note what else you can do to make it healthier for you.

If you live with other people explain the problem carefully to them and gain their cooperation. Be patient with their mistakes and try to keep one room strictly free from pollution, preferably where no one else enters, so that you can retire to it sometimes.

## THE BEDROOM

The bedroom should be very simple and well ventilated. Only keep in those items that are really necessary. Do not have a television set there. It may be wise not to have other electrical equipment in the room either.

## TOILET PREPARATIONS

Most people could get by using far, far fewer personal toiletries than they do. In the Second World War, when I was a child, even soap was in short supply so we had to use it carefully. There were some shampoos and toothpaste but that was about all there was. But we got by with good personal hygiene. I do not remember anyone smelling unpleasantly. It was well after the war that the advertisement with the slogan, "Even your best friend won't tell you", made everyone worried about the possibility of something termed BO and they turned anxiously to deodorants and antiperspirants which I believe were little known of previously (see below).

Even if it causes you no apparent problem only use any chemical substance when absolutely necessary and then use as little as possible. Obviously items marketed as "hypo-allergenic" and "perfume-free" are where to start. But unfortunately "perfume-free" does not always mean free of substances like formaldehyde. Strong artificial chemicals kill our natural bacterial flora allowing the undesirable odour-producing ones to proliferate so making the problem worse rather than lessening it.

## TOOTHPASTE

Some people use baking soda for cleaning their teeth or toothpaste sold by a health food shop. Any form of toothpaste needs to be used in the smallest quantity and rinsed well from the mouth afterwards. (If water is ever rationed we will need to be granted some extra for this and the general necessity to keep pure.) My hygienist was so aghast at me using a toothpaste lacking fluoride that I think that may need to be considered. Do not soak your dentures in chemicals. Clean them with your toothpaste and rinse them well. Keep them in clean water in a clean container overnight.

## SOAP

Use a simple non-perfumed kind and rinse well.

## DEODORANTS

Many of us have a problem with other people's deodorants and deodorants have been accused of causing cancer of the breast. Most of the time good hygiene should suffice but on the occasions that one is in close proximity to others in hot surroundings look for something from the hypo-allergenic ranges like *Dove* or *Simple*. For regular use some people use an alum preparation which is in crystalline form obtainable from Holland and Barrett.

## HAND CREAM

This is needed sometimes especially in cold weather. Ordinary household butter is pure grease and I sometimes use it if I know I will not need to touch anything for a time. But it will result in grease marks on anything touched and a non-perfumed hand cream such made by Simple Health and Beauty Limited will be preferred by most. But, again, use sparingly.

## SHAMPOO

Again choose a simple non-perfumed type in the smallest amount to be effective and rinse well. Do you need to wash your hair so often?

## CONDITIONER

Is it necessary?

## TALCUM POWDER

Use a thick absorbent towel well and it should not be needed. My great-grandmother, so I am told, would cut up old potatoes and leave them in water until a white silt formed on the bottom of the container. She would then pour off the water and dry this deposit and use it as baby powder. If talcum is needed it may be worth trying this.

## SUNSCREEN

Look for a non-perfumed hypo-allergic brand like *Clinique*. Wash it off as soon as it is no longer required. Some authorities say that sunscreen does not affect the role of the skin in producing vitamin D but others say that it does. Until this is resolved perhaps it is prudent to have ten to twenty minutes in the sun to make at least some vitamin D before applying the sunscreen. But avoid exposure when the sun is at its hottest at midday.

## COSMETICS

These were once the province of the better off but they became affordable and had become popularised by the influence of the cinema during the first half of the twentieth century. But they were frowned on by some of the older generation, even then, as it was thought that a made up woman might not have serious attitude to her work. Fashions and thinking change. Personally I would advocate never using any cosmetics at all and that certainly includes hair dye, any other substance applied to the hair or skin and nail varnish. Do not have your hair "permed", or use anything on it but shampoo or some natural substance.

## PERFUMES

They are our major problem. Even if you have one that you are confident does you no harm and you wear it, you will confuse others whom you may have asked not to wear theirs in your presence. How do you know it is so safe?

## VISITORS AND CALLERS

If you know anyone is to visit your home tactfully ask them not to wear perfume or use aftershave or deodorant. Spray deodorants are the worst and sometimes discrete roll-on types may cause no problem. It depends on your level of sensitivity. Even when people comply with your requirements they may smell from the detergent in which their clothes have been washed or just because these modern chemical perfumes persist and adhere to clothes, skin and hair from previous applications. Be ready with your mask. Some people have a sign by their front door instructing people not to enter if they are wearing perfume. Stand firm and do not be intimidated. Do not let anyone in who is likely to make you ill unless it is absolutely necessary. Some make visitors change into special clothes before they enter. It sounds extreme but it may be necessary for the severely affected. If someone is coming to stay with you it must be on condition that they comply with your requirements so tell them about these clearly from the outset. I always ask people to use the toilet preparations that I provide in my bathroom. Of course, no one should ever smoke in your home.

# CLEANING WITHOUT HARMFUL CHEMICALS

An excellent way of cleaning and disinfecting many surfaces is steam. Use a steam cleaner if you can get one. Read the instructions carefully and follow them exactly. One is excellent for the kitchen and the bathroom and larger ones can be used to clean carpets and upholstery. I have even steam-cleaned a teddy bear with one successfully.

But failing that, much dirt can be removed from most surfaces with a clean, damp cloth. Pat or wipe dry with a soft towel for a good finish. Microfibre cloths are excellent and worth investing although do not forget that discarded T-shirts, towels and other absorbent cotton textiles can be cut up and used as dusters and cleaning cloths.

For the more robust surfaces scrubbing brushes or sometimes plastic and stainless steel saucepan scourers and pumice can be substituted for commercial chemicals.

You may be able to tolerate using a washing-up liquid designed for sensitive skin, such is available at Boots, for cleaning. Wear rubber gloves if you can. Always rinse the hands well after contact with any chemical and wash your hands well after wearing rubber gloves. The moisture on their insides that has been given off by your hands makes an attractive environment for germs which you need to avoid transferring to food. Keeping them on a stand such as those sold by Lakeland Plastics when not in use will help the interiors to dry. But putting each losely over a tall empty bottle is just as good.

The dishcloth can be the most dangerous thing in a kitchen. If left damp and screwed up it, too, is an ideal place for germs to flourish. So rinse it well after use and put it somewhere where it will dry – again an empty bottle on the windowsill will do for this – and boil it daily.

I hesitate to say this to people likely to be afflicted with fatigue but old fashioned "elbow-grease" is also an aid to cleanliness. However, the plastic nets in which fruit and similar are sometimes sold make good "scrubbers" for sinks, baths and similar. They can be thrown away as soon as soiled; saving your energy but having been recycled too.

## VACUUMING

Avoid perfume being put into your vacuum cleaner. If the bags are changed according to the instructions it should not smell. Brushing raises dust but vacuuming and damp dusting cut down the amount of dust circulating in the air which is not only better for health but also keeps a room cleaner for longer.

## MISCELLANEOUS CLEANING HINTS

A cut lemon and elbow-grease are said to clean silver. Sodium bicarbonate (baking soda) and also vinegar can be used for a number of cleaning and also laundry purposes.

Vinegar has a degree of disinfectant properties and also can be used to remove spots from stainless steel. Added to the laundry it is said to brighten colours and prevent them from running, as well as whitening whites and fading perspiration stains. It can improve the result of washing floors, countertops and windows. Rubbing carpets with a cloth soaked in a vinegar and water solution may brighten them up if faded. Carpets can be shampooed with a cup of vinegar in five litres of water applied with a soft brush. White vinegar would be preferable for this. Test in an out of the way area first as some carpet dyes run. A solution of half water and half vinegar used to wipe down the area that they walk on can deter ants.

A cupful of vinegar boiled in the kettle can loosen limescale there. Rinse and boil again with plain water which is then discarded.

Boiling vinegar can cut the smell of a drain if left in it for ten minutes before the drain is used.

Glass, including windows and mirrors, can be cleaned with two tablespoons of vinegar added to a small bucket of warm water.

A cupful of sodium bicarbonate followed by a cupful of vinegar poured down the sink can prevent and perhaps clear blockages. Leave for half an hour before flushing with hot water to finish the job.

Vinegar and salt mixed together can be used to clean brass. Sodium bicarbonate can be used to clean the oven. A thick paste of it is smeared over the inside and left overnight before removal. It can also be used to clean hobs and worktops. But remove well from plastic surfaces which it may damage. (Toothpaste containing sodium bicarbonate pitted a plastic washbasin in my house.) Sprinkle sodium bicarbonate on limescale and then spray with vinegar. The foam will loosen it for you to scrub off. Sometimes vinegar alone is sufficient for this task.

Tea and coffee stains can be removed by rubbing a paste of sodium bicarbonate and water on them.

Food spilt in the oven whilst cooking is easier to remove on cooling if it has been sprinkled with salt at the time. Similarly red wine stains are lessened if salt is sprinkled on them immediately the wine is spilt.

Borax can be used to clean the toilet bowl.

## DISHWASHING

Wear gloves (see above) and use a very little hypo-allergenic washing-up liquid with water as hot as you can stand. To remove any food which has dried and stuck on, soak in plain water beforehand and use mechanical means such as saucepan scrubbers, plastic for preference. Rubbing with sodium bicarbonate (baking soda) is a good way to remove tea and coffee stains from china (see above).

AWAYS RINSE ITEMS WELL after using washing-up liquid. Other nationalities quail at the sight of the British washing up in a profuse foam of detergent then immediately wiping the items in a tea towel that soon becomes too heavily impregnated with washing-up liquid itself to remove any from the surfaces. Well-rinsed crockery can be stacked and left to dry. But you may prefer still to dry glass and metal objects. I cannot substantiate this but it used to be said that detergent damaged the lining of the stomach. But we do have quite a lot against the chemicals in detergents anyway (see above). Rinse it away. Stains on the inside of saucepans can be removed by boiling discarded pieces of rhubarb in them.

# LAUNDRY

Items soaked in plain water the night before washing release their dirt more easily thus needing less detergent (and elbow-grease if they are washed by hand). Borax can be added to the soaking water. Look for a hypo-allergenic laundry detergent such as Boots' *Sensitive Skin*. Dry washing out of doors if you can and forget about any fabric conditioner. Sunshine also has a bleaching effect. But if you feel you need a conditioner a pair of Dryer Balls can be used in the dryer (see USEFUL ADDRESSES). These function as mechanical fabric softeners and also aid drying. Iron in a well-ventilated place and be prepared to wear a mask if the heat causes vapours to be given off by the fabric.

One quarter of a cup of lemon juice added to the warm washing water may bleach cotton sheets.

Washing clothes in vinegar or baking soda may remove any smells. But baking soda may cause colours to run.

Vinegar is said to be useful for brightening colours and preventing them from running; also whitening whites and fading perspiration stains. Vinegar may cause corrosion of the metal in a washing machine so use it as a hand wash.

## DRY CLEANING

Avoid having clothing etc. dry-cleaned if possible but if you do, try to keep it to the end of the season so that items can hang for a long time before you need them. Immediately having collected something, outgas it outdoors for a while, if you can, or somewhere like a greenhouse or garage.

Sponging and pressing can sometimes be enough and, best of all, your clothes may be cleaned at home with a steam cleaner. But it is worth looking at labels and buying only those that will wash instead.

## MOTHS

Either horse chestnuts (conkers) or orange peel repel moths if placed in the wardrobe. If using orange peel let it dry first to ensure that it does not grow mould.

## MOULD

This is best prevented, of course, by good ventilation and other means of keeping things dry but black mould, should it occur, on painted plaster, the rubber seals on window frames and on the grouting between bathroom or shower tiles can be treated by bleach. You will need to wear a vapour mask or preferably get someone else to do this. Apply diluted bleach, twice as much water as bleach, and let it dry. Then apply some again and, again, leave to dry naturally.

Ian West of ECOS Organic Paints *The Journal of ACTION Against Allergy* Number 108 (Summer 2013)

## SHOE CLEANING
### *See A SAFE HOME*

## BATHROOMS & SHOWER CUBICLES

Damp areas like these are prime sites for moulds to grow. Unless you have a fan make sure the window is opened for a time after the bath or shower is used. The shower cubicles should be dried after use and the door left open.

The shower head is a site in which disease-causing bacteria can grow. Soak it in warmed white vinegar for twenty minutes every week. This will dissolve any lime deposit as well as killing the bacteria.

## LESSENING SOILING

Obviously if outdoor shoes are removed at the door, floors stay cleaner.

An extractor fan sited near to the hob and running each time you cook will not only improve air quality but walls and surfaces of your kitchen will be freer of grease.

Spills and splashes are easier to clean when dealt with straight away. Try to clean frequently so dirt is easier to remove.

Use a vacuum cleaner rather than a brush to limit circulating dust and pollen.

Look to cook in as few saucepans as you can to save effort. Many things can be doubled up e.g. boiled vegetables. Look for other ways to keep things cleaner but still avoid effort.

## VENTILATION

This is very important indeed. Open your windows as much as you can at every opportunity. But unless one can be sure of being safe from intruders it may be best not to leave one open for more than a few minutes if no one is in the room. In our house we have a system of hanging markers on the doors of rooms in which a window is open so that we do not forget to shut them.

In cold weather open the window whilst you are moving round, such when making the bed or cleaning. Also open windows when you have your outdoor clothing on, either before going out or on coming in. A short burst of cold air has little effect on the temperature of the room as much heat is held in the furniture and furnishings. But it will do you good provided you can keep warm. If you can open windows at the front and back at the same time to create a through draught for a few minutes that will help to disturb pockets of stale air.

It is best to sleep with a window open. But if you live near a busy road or other sources of pollution, open windows on the opposite side of your house or flat and in the least polluted part of the day. The worst pollution on roads is at ground level so upper windows and skylights are usually the best to open. As stale, hot air rises opening windows at the top is best anyway. The old fashioned sash windows are good for this. It is also possible to adjust these so that they are shut but the bottom half is raised a little so that there is a little gap between that and the top half so air can get through. Some modern windows can be fastened, even locked, with a slight gap between window and frame so air can pass. Many houses have ventilators. Most can be open with no security risk allowing a continuous flow of air. You can make your letter box into a ventilator by propping it open with a cork or similar giving extra ventilation though the whole house.

Unblocked chimneys also work as ventilators. The wind passing over the chimney pot sucks air from it and thus from the room below. Open fires burning below them make this effect even greater and may burn off some of the background pollution from within the building too. However, as we know, open fires in their turn cause pollution in the environment. In very bad weather such as during urban fogs when it seems unwise to open a window, causing air movement within your home will disperse some pockets of pollution. Open inside doors to facilitate air movement. Swinging a door open and nearly closed repeatedly works a bit like a fan.

## FANS

Self-cancelling extractor fans in both toilet and bathroom are a great boon and can cut down condensation as well as sweetening the air. A kitchen extractor fan I have already mentioned. Have all of these if you can. If not, open windows in these rooms conscientiously. We are advised not to cook by gas. If you do, energetic ventilation is necessary. A free-standing fan can be used about the house to dispel air pockets that may harbour vapours or just stale air.

## AIR PURIFIERS

Various air purifiers that suck air in mechanically through activated carbon and discharge it minus various impurities are useful. Make sure the one you choose removes vapours as well as pollen and dust mites. Also check that it will not emit perfume or any other chemicals; filter pads are sometimes perfumed. Refuse them. Make sure it is an air purifier. Some so-called air fresheners claim to purify the air! This they may do but they will also pollute it. You also need to check that the air purifier is suitable for the size of room in which you plan to use it. HEPA filters sound attractive but it is an activated carbon one that you need.

## VENTILATION – SUMMARY

Aim for a slow but continuous small stream of air into your home all the time with some greater amount at least once daily. I believe you may find it pays dividends in health. But be aware of the need for security.

## REDECORATING

Aim to have decorating done when the weather allows windows to be open freely. Try to be out of the house whilst this happens but if you must do this yourself wear a strong mask. Try to keep the door of the room closed and the window open during the work. Certainly do not attempt to sleep in the room until all has dried and it feels safe. Make sure that the materials used are the safest for you that you can get (see ADDRESSES).

Wallpaper paste containing antifungal is better avoided. Instead use plain paste and add borax to it. Paint applied over previous paint can cause gases to be released. It is safest to have old painted paper removed and start again from scratch. Unpainted paper can be made easier to strip by adding a generous tablespoon of sodium bicarbonate to a bucket of water or using hot water with vinegar added. We are advised not to use vinyl wallpaper.

A cut onion or some tea bags exposed in a room can remove some of the smell caused by decorating. For furnishings it is best to choose natural fibres as man-made ones tend to give off more toxic gases. New curtains and carpets may need to be allowed to outgas before you can use the room. This may take some time, possibly many months. Getting a friend or relative to vacuum a carpet repeatedly may speed up the process but better still get someone to use a steam cleaner on it. But if you are very lucky just asking the supplier to leave the carpet unrolled during the night before delivery should help. Ask anyway.

Be prepared to allow a newly decorated room to outgas for as long as you can before you use it yourself. Other people using it will speed up the outgassing. One would expect that if one was given samples of carpet etc. to try before purchase, one could ensure that one would be safe with it or not. Unfortunately, as there seems to be an unknown factor often involved in our problem, this would not always work.


## CHOOSING A HOME

Most of us have to try to make the best of the home we have and it is debatable where would be the best place for us to live. Deep in the country, in an isolated spot away from contaminating neighbours, first springs to mind. But that could produce the problems of loneliness, and having to make a long journey to the shops and other facilities may be difficult. Also, rural areas are not always free from pollution: a major trunk road may pass nearby or crops and grassland may be sprayed, droplets spreading on the wind.

A detached house in a quiet side road within walking distance of at least some shops is probably preferable: one with high green hedges which will protect one from some of the vehicle pollution. Avoid low-lying areas as pollution is likely to concentrate there. Look for a home sited on breezy raised ground away from busy roads and industry. A garden gives access to the outdoors and the possibility of outdoor activity and organically grown produce (see below).

An outdoor building may be used to outgas items and a summer house or caravan afford escape from occasional pollution such as during decorating indoor rooms. Avoid integral garages, as if used, vehicle exhaust may contaminate the living area. If it is necessary to use one the car should be driven not backed in so that the exhaust is directed at the open door.

Newly built houses are often small and close to their neighbours. They will contain a number of modern substances liable to give off vapours. An old house may have been renovated resulting in the same. An older house that has not had work done to it recently may be the best as long as it is suitable in its present state or you are confident that you can get it altered safely. We are advised to avoid gas for heating and cooking. Underfloor heating is best avoided too.

## MAKING DO WITH WHAT WE HAVE
*See A SAFE HOME*

## OUTGASSING

Over a period of time objects and substances give off fewer and fewer vapours. But this may take a long time and during this they need to be exposed to the atmosphere. We cannot afford to have them round whilst this happens and want to speed up the process of making them safe if possible.

### Clothing
Wash new clothing as many times as necessary to make it give up its vapours; hanging items outdoors or in an outdoor building is an easy way for some items, such as clothing that cannot be washed, but it is slower. If this is not appropriate or possible, having a room indoors that you do not generally use, in which you can leave things to outgas, is a great boon.

### Various
Wiping some other items with a wrung out cloth that has been dipped in water to which sodium bicarbonate has been added may help where appropriate.

### Glossy paper

I made an outgassing chamber for magazines in a portable metal filing cabinet. In it I have a sheet of activated carbon really intended for deodorising dustbins. The magazines are hung over the rails of the cabinet. Having shut the lid I rock it to and fro to open the pages and leave it for at least a week. Of course, getting other people to read glossy paper publications first may sometimes be sufficient (if they are not themselves disseminators).

### Birthday and Christmas cards

Those you are going to send can be bought ahead of time and outgassed before you handle them by standing them open in the room you do not use. Do the same with those you receive before displaying them.

### New books

Place something between the first two pages to keep the book slightly open and leave it for twenty-four hours preferably in a room you are not using. Move on to the next two pages the next day and so on through the whole book. This takes time. Better let a trusted friend read it first.

### Cars and suitcases

Both should be left closed up out in direct sunshine on a hot day for as long as the sun is on them. The heat will cause gases to be given off more speedily into the interior. As soon as the sun begins to go open them wide to allow the gases to escape. You may prefer to allow someone else to do this for you. Repeat as necessary.

### Hand luggage

This may be treated as suitcases or left open somewhere to gradually outgas. After outgassing your hand luggage, use it outdoors for a short trial period.

### Shoes

Leave to outgas where appropriate and wear out of doors for short periods until safe.

### Second-hand items

Because they have already been used one might think they would be safe. This may be so. But they may be heavily impregnated with other people's perfumes etc. Get someone to choose for you carefully and wash, clean or outgas them according to your specifications.

## GENERAL HEALTH

You have a big enough problem without any more. Try to keep as healthy as you can. Do all you have been brought up to do in that respect. Particularly, as I said earlier, always wash your hands not only before eating but immediately you get in after being out as viruses and other microorganisms can live on surfaces for long periods so you may never have seen the person from whom you caught flu but who left the infection on a door handle which you later touched.

When out and about, if you are unable to use the soap provided, carry a little of your own. Soap is likely to be effective against the germs you may have picked up, even the dreaded Norwalk virus. If you are not severely affected by MCS and it is also possible to hold your breath whilst washing your hands, you may be able to use soap provided if you rinse your hands repeatedly afterwards.

## FOOD

I am not a qualified dietician but I will make some remarks. Beware of those advocating certain types of diet especially crank ones. They may make your nutritional limitations much worse unnecessarily. You need a well-balanced normal diet as far as you can. If you require guidance look for a generalised textbook on basic nutrition written for health professionals.

## TEETH

Having the right amount of the right food is paramount to all life. The beginning of digestion is mastication or chewing. To be able to choose wisely from the range of foods available, to obtain a well-balanced diet and digest it, it is essential to have an effective set of teeth, either natural ones or dentures. But the National Health Service, despite various governments, is no longer providing a free and universally available dental service to all who need it. To me this is highly illogical and, of course, is likely to affect most, those, who through no fault of their own, suffer from an environmental illness preventing them from earning sufficient to pay for private treatment. As good dentition is important it is worth cutting down in other areas of expenditure if one is faced with paying for it. It should be unnecessary to state the importance of close attention to daily dental hygiene (see above). But going to a dentist's surgery is a hurdle to overcome (see TRAVEL). Ask if you can visit the consulting room to see if it affects you before making an appointment and also to talk to the dentist about your condition. Like doctors, some will understand, others will not. I have met both.

## ALLERGIES AND INTOLERANCES

I have not encountered anyone with MCS who has not also some food allergies or intolerances. There are plenty of books on the subject that will guide you in finding out about these. Keeping a detailed diary of what you eat and the symptoms you suffer can help to identify the culprits. Be wary of persons and private clinics that promise to do this for you. They may mean well but some are unreliable. With luck, your GP can refer you to a NHS allergy clinic for this and advice on MCS. Don't forget, that initially at least, when you are avoiding foods you know to be harmful you should avoid others in the same family. For example if milk is your problem, also avoid yoghurt and cheese, cream and butter and anything else containing milk at first. This can be challenged with care later.

If you need to avoid some common foodstuffs you may be missing out on important nutrients. If you suspect this or are not sure, with luck you may be referred to a NHS dietician who will guide you. If not again a textbook on basic nutrition for health professionals from your local library should help. Working alone try to keep an open mind as you are likely to make some mistakes. But be encouraged that after years of abstinence you may find that you can tolerate small amounts of the incitants occasionally again.

## SOME GENERAL COMMENTS ON DIET

Develop a habit of reading all food labels. Items to avoid:

1. Foods with which you know you have problems
2. Foods that you suspect until you find them to be safe

3. Additives
4. Colourings
5. Preservatives
6. Refined carbohydrates like white flour
7. Sugar as much as possible (see SWEETENERS)
8. Artificial sweeteners
9. Processed meat and fish, this includes smoked items
10. All other processed foods where possible
11. Trans-fats and hydrogenated fat; saturated fat should be limited
12. Strictly speaking we should probably avoid alcohol (see SOFT DRINKS AND ALCOHOL) but an occasional small glass of wine may "gladden the heart"
13. We are advised to limit salt intake but do not try to cut it out completely. If you feel particularly tired in hot weather it may help to temporarily have a little more salt. Using iodised salt is advisable. But consult a doctor first if you have any problem associated with your thyroid gland.

## SWEETENERS

Pure white sugar has been highly refined and provides calories but nothing else. Avoid it. It is blamed for the rise of obesity and diabetes in our society. If sweetening is needed unpasteurised honey is probably the best choice for adults. Although it is not safe for the very young it contains phosphorus and potassium and has other good properties. Next in the line is normal commercially produced honey. Then comes cane molasses which seems to contain some beneficial substances including minerals beside just sugar and has a strong taste that is likely to limit quantities used. If sugar is required look for raw cane sugar and note that some brown sugars are white sugar to which a little molasses has been added to colour them. Choose cane sugar which is likely to have been produced using fewer chemicals than that from sugar beet.

Dried fruit, especially dates, make healthier sweeteners for cakes, puddings and breakfast cereals than processed sugar as they contain the natural sugar, fructose. But it is still wise to avoid sweet things if you can. Flavouring food with cinnamon can make it seem sweeter.

## THE IDEAL DIET

The ideal diet is probably one close to Dr Mackarness's "Stone Age Diet" in that he advocated fresh meat, poultry and fish, well balanced by fresh fruit and vegetables, with filtered or spring water, herbs, teas, olive oil and fresh nuts. But most of us will want to add food made from grains and it now seems that red meat should be limited. Until recent history grain would have always meant good nutritious wholegrain. Wholegrains are good sources of B-group vitamins. Those particularly worried about pesticides are best advised to have wholegrains which are grown organically. If possible have home-made bread. A bread-making machine is a boon and ideal for this and for avoiding additives. Although organic food is probably best it is difficult to insist on and expensive. But growing your own, unless it is in an area of pollution is an excellent occupation.

## MEAT AND OTHER PROTEIN

Red meat is an important source not only of protein but iron and other minerals and vitamins. However, too much is not good and we are advised not to eat more than 500g cooked weight of red meat a week. That is equal to 700 to 750g when raw. Protein can be provided instead by poultry, fish, cheese, dried beans, peas and lentils, eggs and also nuts and seeds. These latter offer a number of nutritional benefits but when eating peas, beans and lentils, known collectively as pulses, have some bread or other grain food with them so as to obtain all of the essential amino acids.

## FISH

Fish should be a good source of good nutritious protein and we are encouraged to eat oily fish.

However, they can live in polluted water and can concentrate pollutants into their bodies. Shellfish and types of fish that live on the bottom of the sea are most at danger of doing this. Fish, such as salmon and trout which are farmed, are subjected to chemicals such as anti-fungals in their water. Salmon whose flesh looks the brightest orange may have been fed dye to make it so. So we must balance this against the likely health benefits.

Until better advice is available I suggest fish not more than twice a week and salmon, as advised to pregnant women, not more than three times a year. Small fish, such as sprats, are likely to be less polluted than those larger ones that have concentrated pollution in a chain of large eating smaller. Shark has recently been said to contain high levels of mercury and flatfish, which live at the bottom of the ocean, are quite liable to have absorbed pollution too.

## FRUIT AND VEGETABLES

It is recommended that fruit and vegetables should make up one third of the daily diet. Try to have some green vegetable every day as the chlorophyll will bind with toxins in the gut so that they are expelled. Vary these, as too much cabbage can prevent iodine absorption whilst too much spinach may prevent iron being absorbed. Winter lettuce has been linked to high pesticide loads. Lettuce has a low nutritional value. Shredded cabbage and grated carrots make a good winter salad. Mustard and cress can be grown on your kitchen windowsill like you did at school. Vegetables are generally preferable to fruit in being lower in sugar content and by taking a variety of colours one will help provide trace nutrients. Root vegetables are generally cheap and can taste nicer if mashed. Beetroot, usually thought of for salads, can be eaten roasted. It is useful in enhancing the colours of red lentils or as an inclusion in any other stew or casserole and there is, of course, always borscht. Beetroot is said to prevent high blood pressure. Onions are believed to help prevent clotting in the blood vessels.

Do not be too hooked on potatoes. Vary your carbohydrates with rice, barley and other grains. As these do not provide the little vitamin C that potatoes do, make sure to have fresh vegetables in the same meal. When choosing fruit, note that grapes are likely to be the most contaminated with pesticide residues. Strawberries, although they have good food value, may also be high in pesticides too. Probably this is most likely out of season. It has recently been suggested that those with a tendency to depression may do well to limit their fruit intake as well as that of sugar and other carbohydrates.

## MILK AND MILK PRODUCTS

Milk is a good source of calcium well known to be needed for healthy bones and it is also important for other aspects of good health. If you do not take milk it is probably advisable to take a calcium supplement or use an artificial milk such as soya milk to which calcium has been added. Milk made from almonds, hazelnuts or rice is also available. Although these are processed foods their usefulness may outweigh this consideration. Cheese is a good source of protein as well as of calcium. Live yoghurt is good for gut health. If you have a problem with candida and wish to avoid milk sugars or you cannot take milk at all, capsules containing the same bacteria can be obtained from a health-food shop. Those who cannot take milk may find that they can tolerate either butter or cheese as the milk sugar lactose may be their problem. A little butter may be preferable to margarine which is a processed foodstuff and may contain something you prefer to avoid.

## COOKING

If you are lucky you will be able to cook your own food or have someone cook it for you to your specifications. Even if you are tired it is a good thing to cook your own as you will know what it contains. But you may need to start in a small way and gradually do more as things improve for you. Culinary herbs, also spices, make good flavourings and may have some health benefits too.

Cloves may also discourage candida. They can be added to soups, stews and casseroles as well as fruit dishes. Use a pinch of ground cloves in dishes from which they could not be easily removed before serving. Thyme has antiseptic properties. Crumble a sea kelp tablet into savoury dishes as a way to ensure enough iodine is taken but do not if you or anyone eating it has any problem with the thyroid gland, without taking medical advice first.

Regard garlic as a friend. Eaten raw the crushing between the teeth converts the alliin to allicin which makes the blood less likely to clot. Garlic lowers the cholesterol and has anti-inflammatory and anti-viral properties. To use in cooking crush and leave for a few minutes before use. It is also good against candida. If raw garlic seems repulsive, bury pressed garlic in bread and butter or margarine. Garlic does stay on the breath so eat it at times when you are unlikely to be about to meet other people.

## BREAKFAST

Breakfast should be substantial enough to see you through the morning so that you do not fall to the temptations of biscuits and sticky buns. It is advised that breakfast should constitute 20% of the daily calorie count. Choose wholegrain non-sugared cereals such as puffed wheat, shredded wheat or unsweetened muesli. You can mix up your own muesli from porage oats, nuts and dried fruit. Cut up some fresh fruit on it before you eat it. Porage itself is wholesome and also warm. It is best made from oatmeal but porridge oats are quicker and easier. Use low-fat milk or fruit juice on it. If you really need a sweetener use dried or stewed fruit.

We are now told that we do not absorb cholesterol from eggs and so a boiled or scrambled egg or two can be consumed in the morning. My recent reading suggests this may be a good thing. After all, eggs, as do seeds, contain all the required constituents for the formation of a new individual. Some of those who have a problem with eggs may be able to tolerate them if they hard-boil them or eat only the yolk.

## SMALL APPETITE

If your appetite is small be careful, nevertheless, to have a mixed and healthy diet but just cut down on amounts. Have portions the size you require. If you have to buy large amounts but live alone try to freeze half.

# HEALTH FOODS

Remember that so-called health foods are not always healthy options. If you prepare and cook your own food you will know what it contains.

# FOOD PREPARATION

Prepare food carefully. Wash meat and fish under cold water taking care not to splash. Wash your hands and wash everything that has been in contact with raw meat and fish in hot water straight away after handling them. Fruit and vegetables may have been sprayed so wash and then rinse them twice. Keep a bowl especially for this alone. The bowl will need washing but rinse it free of traces of washing-up liquid afterwards.

Wash apples, pears and everything that can be peeled and then peel before eating. Do not scrape carrots. Peel them thickly even if organically produced. After repeatedly washing Brussels sprouts, cabbages, kales, broccoli and cauliflower cover with boiling water and cook rapidly as usual. But dispose of the water as pesticides will have leached into it. It has been rumoured that some vegetable producers grow produce for their own use separately from the commercial crops.

If cooking potatoes in their skins scrub very well first but do not eat the skins. Insist that food preparation areas are kept free from all chemicals and do not let people put other items on them.

## FOOD STORAGE

For most people it is impossible to have fresh food all the time, although aim to do so as much as you can. Food should, of course, be stored according to the instructions that come with it. Glass, being inert, makes the best containers both for cupboards and the fridge but do not buy special ones where glass jam jars will do.

Wax cartons, if they are available, are probably advisable for freezing food. But if you need to use polythene bags and boxes in the freezer remove the food from them as soon as possible after getting it out. Do not use plastic crockery at home as the surface easily becomes roughened encouraging germs to grow. Plastic food and drink containers have been found not to be as dangerous as they were rumoured to be but if heating food in plastic in the microwave do so strictly according to the instructions that come with it. It would still be sensible to part with any plastic containers and crockery that you have had for some time as they may date from a time when manufacturers were less careful about phthalates, and all plastic containers should be replaced frequently.

Tinned food is best avoided and certainly transfer any food not used immediately straight from the tin into glass containers and put in the fridge. Aluminium foil is suitable for wrapping bland items like bread and perhaps meat but do not get salt on it (see SAUCEPANS ETC. below). It takes a toll on the environment so please wash it and put it out for recycling after use.

*Cancer Research UK* (16 March 2010)


# SAUCEPANS ETC

For cooking, heat-resistant glass is best because it is inert. Glass saucepans can be obtained. But after these, stainless steel ranks next. Lined and enamelled vessels are best avoided. They can peel and chip. Aluminium can leach out into acidic foods cooked in aluminium pans. Examples of this are rhubarb, fruits and pickles. Highly salted food causes pitting of aluminium containers. Although I do not advise that everyone should rush out and buy a new set of saucepans it may be wise to phase out aluminium ones as quickly as you can. Ideally, food and drink should be taken from glass too. It is certainly sensible to eat acidic food from glass dishes as acid can leach the lead from lead silicate in the glaze of ceramics into the food.

Lecture with demonstration to *Get Lead out of Petrol* workshop by Professor Bryce Smith, (27th March 1982)

## DIETARY SUPPLEMENTS

It seems likely that most of us with MCS need some extra vitamins above that which the diet provides and probably minerals too. This is generally advised. At present it is a difficult topic because too much of anything is a bad thing and how much any individual needs varies so it is difficult to advise on amounts. The Recommended Daily Allowance has often been criticised as too low. I believe this may most likely be true for us. Halibut or cod liver oil and vitamin C or, better still, a good quality multi-vitamin and mineral supplement are, I think, likely to be a wise choice but do not take one containing iron. Iron deficiency should be diagnosed and treated by a doctor of medicine.

There is a suggestion that we may be deficient in some of the B group vitamins, vitamins $B_5$ and $B_{12}$ in particular. Brewer's yeast provides this group all in the correct balance except $B_{12}$ in which it is deficient. Brewer's yeast is easily obtained from health-food shops and pharmacies and also is fairly cheap. Vitamin $B_{12}$ is found in liver, beef, pork, eggs, milk, cheese and kidney. A health professional may advise supplement of a particular B group and it is likely that a supplement of vitamin $B_{12}$ may be useful. If taking individual vitamins of the B group unsupervised it may be wise to do so only for short periods as this may cause an imbalance in the others.

At the time of writing, vitamin D has emerged out of obscurity and its benefits are being acknowledged. Many of us get little opportunity to be in the sun however. Oily fish, another good source of vitamin D, may be contaminated by polychlorinated biphenyls and dioxins★ and it is recommended that women and girls (and possibly men if affected by MCS) should not eat more than two 140g portions a week. So if you are not taking a multi-vitamin supplement it may be wise discussing a vitamin D supplement with your doctor. If you are housebound or otherwise getting little sun ask if you need more than even a multi-vitamin supplement may supply.

★Dioxin contamination is hopefully declining.

## WATER AND BEVERAGES

Taking an adequate amount of water each day is extremely important. We are advised that we need between a litre and a half and two litres of water a day; the most, of course, when in hot buildings or during hot weather. We probably get about four hundred millilitres from our food. The best way to judge if one is drinking enough is to look at the colour of one's urine. It should be a light straw colour. If it is darker more fluid is required. Too light a colour indicates too much is being drunk. For us, plenty of fluid is important to make sure as many toxins are excreted as possible. Water alone in too much quantity can pall. But it can be taken as tea or coffee or flavoured with fruit juice.

Coffee is pleasant and may have some beneficial properties but the amount daily should be limited probably to one or two cups. An excess of coffee can make one pass too much urine and also cause tenseness and insomnia. The habit of drinking at least some plain water each day is a good one. Some people drink distilled water to avoid all chemicals. However, this may mean that they do not get some of the "good" chemicals in the water such as silica. Filtering your own tap water is more convenient and preferable to buying mineral waters which vary and mostly have to be obtained in plastic bottles, glass ones being expensive.

## SOFT DRINKS AND ALCOHOL

Commercial soft drinks tend to contain a lot of sugar plus chemical ingredients and are best avoided. We have always known that too much alcohol is bad for one. Also it contains sugar but taken occasionally and in small amounts it can be pleasurable and sociable. It would be most unwise for us to exceed the recommended amounts of units*. Also one often does not know what

*I am confused as to what may be safe for the general population. Cancer Research UK says less than three units a day for a man and less than two for a woman. The Government says up to no more than four units and two to three respectively. Ideally, as I have said, perhaps we with MCS should have none. Red wine is supposed to have health benefits such as reducing bad cholesterol. At present each must draw their own conclusion.

the ingredients are. Beers approved by the Campaign for Real Ale are brewed with traditional ingredients, as also are some ciders. But other ciders may have colourings added. Some producers of both these drinks give a customer care telephone number on their bottles and are willing to discuss ingredients. Most wines carry a warning about sulphites but no declaration that there are no other chemicals in them. Bear in mind that alcohol can cause you to be short of water.

## CANDIDA

It is extremely common for those suffering from MCS to also suffer from an overgrowth of the fungus once called *Monilia albicans* and now known as candida. It is normally found in the gut and on the skin of human beings and this presents a problem. Unless it shows itself as thrush that is creamy white spots in the mouth or a creamy white discharge somewhere else it is difficult to show that there is an overgrowth.

Overgrowth of candida in the gut, also called "candidiasis" can result in "bloatedness", diarrhoea and or constipation, an itch around the anus and flatulence (wind). It can cause damage to the gut wall leading to food allergies and migraines and is also associated with brain fog. It can also disrupt the functioning of the endocrine system resulting in a number of symptoms and also affect the immune system. At present it is not known what a normal level of candida in the gut is and what level constitutes an overgrowth. So measurements cannot be taken. But I understand work is being done on this.

Candida is a big subject and I advise those who think they are affected to discuss this with their doctor initially. There are a number of books on the subject often under the heading "gut dysbiosis". The National Candida Society is a source of information and advice. However, I will say:

1. Before beginning an anti-candida regime, think ahead and plan carefully; it is not easy and needs to be followed for six to eight months continuously.
2. Avoid metal dental fillings.
3. Include plenty of the Brassica family in your diet straight away. These include cabbage, turnip, broccoli, Brussels sprout, radish, mustard shoots and cauliflower. Use lots of garlic, taking it raw is best, and also cloves and onion.

## MISCELLANEOUS

## BRAIN FOG AND LETHARGY

These certainly slow one up. Take them into account when making plans. Do everything when you are at your brightest as early as you can. Do not leave things to the night before they are needed. Try to have adequate sleep.

## IRRITABLE BOWEL SYNDROME

The discomfort can sometimes be relieved by sipping a little whisky diluted with tonic water. Dolomite tablets may provide some general help but please read the caution on calcium in the sleep section. This is a recognised medical condition and should be diagnosed and treated by a doctor.

## DRY, BLOCKED NOSE

A dry, inflamed and painful blocked nose can be relieved by steam inhalations. Small handheld steam inhalers can be obtained from pharmacies. If the nose is seriously blocked adding a very small menthol crystal to the water will clear it so that the beneficial steam can reach all the mucosa. It is important to get your nose as clear so that the gases which are affecting you are not retained in your sinuses. A soothing effect can be obtained by adding a few drops of compound of benzoin co (*Friars Balsam*) to the water instead. The water needs to be just below boiling and will be very hot so handle the inhaler carefully. Stay in the same room until your nose has cooled down to normal afterwards. When out and about or during the night a *Vicks* inhaler may give some help. Or try sniffing some *Vicks* vapour rub on a handkerchief. It is important to breathe through your nose as much as possible. Walking in the cold air and concentrating on breathing through the nose helps. Do all you can to prevent yourself having to breathe through your mouth all the time.

## GOING OUT AND EXERCISE

Do not let this condition make you a couch potato. Do all you can to resist becoming housebound. Daily exercise is important even though it may present difficulties. If you are not in the habit of exercising it is prudent to check with your doctor before you start as of course you must if you suffer from some other condition. Some exercise can be taken at home. An exercise bicycle or other apparatus may be useful but not important and may be a bit ambitious if you are very unfit when you start. Even going up and down stairs a few times a day more than normal will help. There are various charts and other advice available in the media and books on schemes of exercises for indoors.

But try, if you can, to get out into the open air even on days when you find it difficult. A short, brisk walk before breakfast is ideal. The cold air is beneficial to the nose. However, this may be unrealistic to you. If so, decide on a time that the air is likely to be less polluted, probably after the morning rush but before the afternoon school run and evening rush. Choose the quietest roads. The middle of a public park should be pleasant with low pollution but look out for grass spraying or similar activities. Walking in the country can be delightful but look out for and avoid crop spraying. Always keep a protective mask at the ready.

You may find it possible to use a gym although some are heavily polluted by air fresheners. Ring up first and ask where they are. If they are only in the changing room and you live nearby you may do as I have done and go dressed ready and come home to shower so avoiding using them. Find out when the quietest period is so that it will be easier to avoid disseminators.

Swimming would be excellent were it not for the changing-room situation and the chlorinated water. For those who can take the risk it might be worth examining the possibility of using an outdoor pool. Some pools may sterilize their water with a method other than chlorine. If this is with ozone, that itself could be an irritant, but it could be worth finding out although be prepared to be disappointed.

Gardening is a good activity providing both fresh air and exercise which can be moderated according to individual needs. Although it is in the nature of things that shrubs sometimes die and crops can fail, over all this can be a very satisfying hobby and a means of obtaining unpolluted food. A garden is a pleasant place to sit. Of course chemical pesticides, weed-killers and other chemicals must be banned. There are ways of overcoming pests naturally, for example growing calendulas (marigolds) can keep aphids from nearby plants.

The amount and nature of the exercise one takes is a very individual thing depending on one's age and physical state. But whatever it is, starting and increasing the amount should be taken gently. Overdoing things may cause harm or, at the best, discouragement. Do not push yourself too hard. Once you have achieved a regular habit you can gradually increase your activity.


## GOING ON HOLIDAY

This is possible if you are not too badly affected. But it is difficult. Some people use a caravan or own a holiday cottage or chalet so that everything can be made to conform to their needs. Although risky, if you are not too seriously affected, it is possible to stay in some hotels if you don't mind wearing a mask in public areas like corridors. Find a hotel with accommodation free for when you want it and ask if they can accommodate your dietary needs. If they can, before booking ask to speak to the head housekeeper on the phone. Explain your room requirements and ask about their use of air fresheners and other items which may be difficult for you. Some will tell you straight out that they could not possible comply with what you want. But sometimes you find someone who will understand the problem and is willing to provide what you need.

Confirm your booking making it clear it is on this understanding and promise a second letter describing your needs in detail to get there about a week before you will arrive. It is also prudent to telephone a reminder to the housekeeper a few days before you go as I have more than once found the letter had become stuck at the reception desk. Make it clear that it is not that you are fussy but that it is an important health issue. Be prepared that you may need to contact a number of hotels before you find a suitable one.

However, this is not safe for someone who is badly affected because, as even with the best will in the world, there can be flaws in the arrangement. I once booked into a very understanding B & B. They had prepared a lovely room and bathroom with no air fresheners, sprays, polishes or disinfectants. But they did their own laundry and the vapours from their detergent and, even worse, fabric conditioner affected me badly despite me using my own sleeping bag and putting the pillow in a plastic bag. The smell hung heavily over everything for all of our stay. I would advise travelling as I do now, with a vapour-proof pillowcase or, better still, your own pillow as well as your sleeping bag.

Although there are many excellent B & B establishments, hotels are the best bet because their laundry arrangements usually do not involve the bedding becoming perfumed as home-washed linen is likely to be. A room that is easily accessed so that you do not need to pass through areas controlled by fire doors where air fresheners may be used is preferable. The window should not open onto an area where swimming pools, exhausts from heating systems and similar are ventilated. Ask for the room window to be left open after preparation to ventilate any perfume from the previous guests. Make sure there will be no chemical hanging in the toilet bowl and no bowl of potpourri in the bedroom.

On arrival open the window wider for a while and run cold water down the wash basin and bath, also flush the toilet. Run the fan for a while if there is one. However, one of the hazards of hotels is that perfume, and even the smoke from illegal smoking, can sometimes enter bathrooms from the ventilation system. It may be necessary to put something along the bottom of the door when you are in the room to cut down on vapours from the corridor.

Disseminators in the dining room are a hazard. But if you are lucky you can ask to change to another table or take your meal on a tray to your room. Most people, when they understand the problem, can be very kind. Avoid relying on room service if you can, not only because of the cost but because of the loss of social stimulus that it would entail. Renew the arrangements each time you go to the same establishment. People forget and staff and managements change. For the same reasons, do not rely on other people's recommendations alone. But if holidaying is becoming too difficult or too expensive for you, sleeping in a different room for a while or even a different way round in the same room can create the sense of a change.

# TRAVEL

Ideally one will be accompanied by someone who knows you and can intercede on your behalf if things get difficult – the articulate advocate. A second person adds weight to what you say. An example was when a waitress was obviously not taking seriously my enquiries about ingredients. A friend in the party intervened firmly, "She gets ill if she eats egg." This was all that was needed and the waitress made off to the kitchen to check ingredients with the chef. Out of kindness and to foster good relations, in those circumstances I usually say, "I would prefer 'x' but to save your legs if you find that has egg in it bring me 'y' instead."

If possible travel at off-peak times when road pollution is lower. Needless to say the car window should stay closed when other traffic is about. Look for quiet places away from main roads when you want to stop. If it has to be a car park, aim for the quietest area. Modern cars with air conditioning are a boon to such as us.

Public transport is less easy but quieter periods give the better chance of moving from disseminators. But go well armed with vapour masks and do not be too embarrassed to use them. Unfortunately the air conditioning can cause problems sometimes (see below). If there is a frequent service and the need is dire one can get off a service bus and wait for the next. On trains, if they are not too crowded, it may be possible to move away from a disseminator. On a coach one is likely to find oneself more constrained. Once when trying to push my boundaries, I had to get the driver to stop and let me off as we approached a motorway when a perfumed air-conditioning system on a coach was threatening to overcome me. I then had to walk back to the last town and seek a bus to take me home. This is not an adventure that I would recommend to others. But if using a bus or coach a seat at the front prevents perfume wafting backwards to you.

Air travel is even more difficult. Apart from perfumes and deodorants from other passengers and possible chemicals in the air conditioning, on some flights insecticide sprays may be used in the cabin. If you have to fly, a good supply of reliable masks is a must. Inform the airline of your problems when you book and ask to be warned when spraying is going to happen so that you can protect yourself as best you can. I have been advised that one should warn the airline on booking that one may require oxygen so that it can be used if things get very difficult. Since my condition has been serious I have only taken internal flights. These have been successful, even pleasant.

## AIR CONDITIONING

Air conditioning in vehicles is a boon but can also be a hazard. When the air conditioning is serviced a disinfectant is used which has a perfume to mask the smell. This contaminates the air for a period when the vehicle returns to use. Unfortunately servicing is likely to go on all the year and it is not usually possible to predict if a recently serviced public vehicle will be used on any particular route. When having a private car serviced specify that no perfume must be added to the air conditioning. To compound matters coaches and taxis are likely to have air fresheners in them also. It may be possible to arrange for an air-freshener-free taxi if it is ordered in advance but this depends on persons being willing and able to cooperate. A single driver owner, however, who does not use them, would be worth seeking out.

## OTHER PEOPLE

We are dependent on the good will of other people that they do not make life any more difficult, perhaps even dangerous, for us than it has to be. Therefore we must maintain cordial relations with them and limit, as much as we can, the effect that our problems have on those around us. Always be grateful for the concessions people make on your behalf. Do not demand them as a right unless they have been agreed in a contract beforehand; for example, as would be in the use of hypo-allergenic materials in house decorating. If being entertained by others, although one has to avoid foods that definitely affect one, concessions should be made out of kindness to the host and so as not to seem too difficult to be invited again.

People come in two groups: those who can understand and believe the reality of MCS and those who do not. With all the publicity allergy now has I think the latter group may be dwindling. I always tell people about the problem as this explains my behaviour in moving away from them, leaving a room, wearing a mask, etc. Although it is not usually MCS, people often recount experience with friends or relatives who have some similar problem. Although not classed as allergy it is useful to use that word with the general public as words like sensitivity and intolerance can be misunderstood and mistaken as mere dislike. Most people know the word "allergy".

Having adequately explained the situation, leave it at that unless it becomes relevant to refer to it. People will tire if they get bulletins on your daily difficulties. Have compassion on those who find the concepts difficult. Be as consistent as you can. For example, about food, people may become confused and doubtful, if knowing yourself that you can tolerate small occasional amounts, you take a little of something you have told them previously that you need to avoid.

Relatives can be difficult. Sometimes it is perhaps that they cannot bear to see what is happening to a loved one so deny the problem is real for their own peace of mind. Sometimes they find the restrictions in the household of someone with MCS just too irksome. Sometimes there are other dynamics in the family situation. Whatever it is, living with someone who has MCS is hard. The worst must be the anxiety if someone is liable to go into anaphylaxis. At best someone with MCS impinges on the normalities of daily life of the other members of the household.

Nevertheless many relatives, such as my husband, are saints. He has been known to sit in a hotel room in his overcoat so that we could have the window open wide, or leave immediately with me, with great patience, because, on arrival somewhere, I could not enter because of an air freshener. There have been many instances like these. Sometimes concerned friends or relatives can seem over protective. One must be patient with this and thankful they are as they are.

# DOCTORS, DENTISTS AND HOSPITALS
*(See also SECTION A – RELATIVES, FRIENDS AND HEALTH PROFESSIONALS)*

Some people are afraid to reveal to health professionals that they have MCS. It is, unfortunately, a decision that we all have to make individually. I would not like to give general advice on this. Ideally one should feel as safe about MCS as one would to admitting to diabetes or arthritis. One of the aims of this booklet is to make everyone aware of the condition as a real, physical illness. It will come, I hope, as it has to other maladies in the past.

Personally I tell everyone because the discomforts and distress I have from time to time suffered have been due to ignorance rather than unkindness or disbelief. Unfortunately communication can be poor in the NHS and one may find that one has to explain MCS to every member of staff separately. This is where the articulate advocate can be a help particularly in emergency admissions when one might be too ill to make a coherent case for oneself.

Once a doctor has accepted that you have MCS ask to have it written on the front of your notes. Wear an identity tag at all times which states that you suffer from Multiple Chemical Sensitivity and have a list of your known incitants in your wallet. Although, as I have said, some people say that they fear that revealing MCS could prejudice attitudes to their other conditions, and I am not able to refute this, mostly I have found health-care professionals kind and understanding, some particularly so. But if you need to wear a mask when meeting a health professional try to make it a coloured one. The white ones look like clinical masks and give a first impression that you are fastidiously fearful of infection and, as well as giving the wrong idea, can irritate.

For a planned admission you can list your needs and discuss them with the staff. Give them a written copy. Some people need to take their own sheets and other items; if this is so this needs to be agreed. You will need a single room with the door clearly labelled that no one should enter wearing perfume or aftershave, or use chemicals, etc. and the window needs to open onto an area of clean air.

Regarding dental treatment, as well as avoiding amalgam, it may be wise to avoid stainless-steel dentures because stainless steel has chrome and other metals in it which could be troublesome to some. Some people advise us to take the very first morning medical and dental appointments so that the consulting rooms have not been contaminated by disseminators. However, there is the likelihood that there will still be fumes from the early morning cleaning.

Also, travelling at that time one will encounter people straight from their morning shower exuding deodorants, etc. Even walking to an early appointment I have found my nose repeatedly thus assaulted. On arrival tell someone about your condition i.e. that you may need to take refuge in the open air, the reason for your mask, etc., as appropriate. Sometimes kindly staff may be able to let you wait in an empty room.

## REST AND SLEEP

It may be that the fatigue and lethargy ensures you have a lot of rest. Rest is important for everyone and one should not feel guilty about taking some rest during the day; although exercise and activity are necessary too. Few people need more than seven to eight hours sleep each night. If one does not feel sleepy during the day it is likely that one is sleeping long enough. But insomnia may be a problem for some people with MCS. If one does not sleep enough at night a cat nap between 1 and 3 p.m. may help. If one is chronically tired twenty-five-minute naps at lunchtime and around 5 or 6 p.m. may help one catch up on lost sleep. The main thing is not to be too anxious about insomnia. If you cannot get to sleep, or wake in the night, try to concentrate on how comfortable it is being in bed but do not think about sleeping and you may. Lying in bed worrying about if one can get to sleep is counterproductive.

It is important, of course, that the bed is comfortable, the room is at the right temperature, and adequately ventilated and quiet. Do not have a heavy meal in the evening, but a small snack of either banana, nuts, tuna, chicken or turkey an hour before bed may help. Simmer down during the evening and do not do anything taxing or exciting before retiring.

A relaxing bath may help and going to bed early with no idea of immediate sleep but a plan for some light, relaxing reading may bring success. Provided one has no kidney or bladder problem then a calcium tablet before bed, or if one wakes in the night, may help. If this leaves you too sleepy in the morning cut it down to half or even a quarter of a tablet. They tend to vary in strength between 100 and 500 mgs. Make sure you have plenty to drink the next morning.

If none of this, or any other practical advice you have been given, works then it is time to ask your doctor for something to help you to sleep. But do not become dependent on it. It is important to get back to sleeping naturally again. Once you have had a series of good nights and feel refreshed try a night without. If it does not work take a pill the next night but after a few nights try without again. If you slept, then try again the next night and so on, just taking a sleeping pill the next night after a bad one until, hopefully, you do not need them anymore. The odd poor night or two from time to time happens to us all. It is when they continue for a prolonged period that it is a problem and can be very, very wearing.

## CHALLENGES – PUSHING ONE'S BOUNDARIES

It's likely that one may be getting frequent proof that one still has a problem with some incitants. However, particularly with items like food, one may find that after a year or two of rigidly avoiding it, one can take a small amount occasionally. Challenges sometimes happen by accident. Planned ones are, of course, safer. But they need careful consideration. Questions to ask oneself are:

- Can I limit this to only a small exposure?
- Is this important enough to be worth trying?
- What is the worst that can happen if I do react?
- Could it be dangerous?
- Will I be able to cope?
- Are the circumstances suitable?
- Is anything planned to happen that will make a reaction too inconvenient?

One successful challenge does not mean that the item has now become safe. Checking will be necessary and increases of exposure must be slow and gradual. As I have said, try not to become housebound. It is very easy not to want to leave the only place you feel safe. The above same questions need to be asked before going somewhere. It is important, of course, to be able to leave immediately if things do go wrong. Those of us who can use vapour masks are luckier when venturing out. Remember that even though you can still smell the perfume it may still withstand the chemical although this cannot always be relied upon. Continuing to wear the mask for a while after one has reached safety may sometimes help (see TRAVEL).

## ELECTRICAL SENSITIVITY

A number of people find they cannot tolerate being near electrical equipment when in use. Although some of these are known to give off ozone there seems to be another factor. Sadly it has not been possible for me to research this but I would suggest it may be something to do with further irritation of already irritated or damaged tissue. A full scientific investigation is needed.

## THE SPIRITUAL DIMENSION

To those of a religious faith I say, "Do not let MCS get between you and your religious practice." It may be easier to go to a place of worship than you think. I speak from an experience that has been mainly Christian but hope that what I say will have equal application to those of other faiths. Churches and chapels and, I suspect, other sacred buildings too, commonly have high roofs and no ceilings so gases easily go upwards and away. Incense can be a problem although attending a service when it is not used may be sufficient for some. Many Anglican and, of course, non-conformist Christian churches do not use it at all. It is usually possible to keep away from disseminator worshippers as churches are rarely full except at major festivals. Try to sit away from other people. Even if you are being shown to a seat it is acceptable to ask to be placed according to your needs.

Explain that you have "allergies". If you think you may need to leave during the service try to be near a door. Do not hesitate to wear a mask if necessary. It is more important that you are there than how you appear to others.

If you cannot get to a place of worship try to do what you can at home with sacred and other books of your religion and the radio and television to live your spiritual life. You may be able to get a minister of religion or an appropriate lay person to visit you at home. Do not be shy of insisting on the need for no perfume, etc. I have similar advice to those who have not previously been involved in religious practice. Please consider exploring it.

Religion has become neglected in the West these days. Partly, I think, because people are unaware that there is a need for it and partly because of the explosion of knowledge over the last two-hundred years. This latter has made it difficult for people to equate what they read and learn with religious belief. Speaking of Christianity as the religion with which I am familiar, I fear that it often seems couched in terms related to a bygone era rather than this one. Religion needs to be presented in a credible way relevant to our present knowledge and understanding. However, it is interesting to note that some scientists state that the marvels they discover strengthen their religious faith rather than weaken it. Scientific knowledge is not as incompatible as some suggest.

Archaeological studies too back up parts of the Bible's narrative. Unfortunately we are educated to look critically at things and for absolute proof whereas spirituality requires a different mindset. You do not need faith to start with but by the grace of God, in time, it may be given to you.

# SUMMARY

There is hope in the future. Some parts of America already have "no-perfume" areas indicating that the problem is not only acknowledged but addressed. There are also communities in the USA of people with MCS living together to maintain a safe environment. At Leimbach, Zurich, some flats have been built to be free of chemicals and electricity. Some Canadian schools are reported to have scent-free or scent-awareness programmes. Staff have observed that perfumes affect concentration. In the autumn of 2012, the European Union proposed rulings limiting the ingredients of perfumes. Hopefully Britain too, like other countries, will officially recognise our condition soon.

Following that there is hope of research and some help for us. Also, as I have said, it seems that some research is being done to discover what normal gut flora is. That, too, could have some relevance on our condition. One can also hope that in due course a more precautious attitude will be taken to chemicals so that mankind can benefit from their use without suffering harm. We know that fish pass the pollution in their bodies along the food chain to larger fish that eat them. Human mothers can pass 25% of the pollutants they have absorbed to their first babies and 20% to the next.

That means that infants can be starting life with a load even before they start absorbing pollutants themselves.

Meanwhile, as individuals, we have to do the best we can for ourselves. After a lifetime of observing people, friends, relations and, in the past, patients suffering from illness or disability, I believe that the most important thing is the individual's attitude. Denial is no use. One must accept the problem and face up to it head on, take full stock of the situation and decide how best to live with it. Although a period of grief for what is lost is probably inevitable, try not to think of what you have lost but what you still can do and that you are going to cope against the odds. Live the life you have to the full. My final words are a consensus of advice from those MCS sufferers I have contacted whilst researching this:

- Avoid chemicals that affect you
- Keep cheerful
- Keep going
- Be self-reliant
- Get plenty of fresh air.

To which I add, "Keep your exposure to other chemicals low but be prepared to make concessions on occasions where others are involved as far as you can".

I hope this booklet has been some help.

# A STORY FOR THOSE WHO ARE STILL "DISBELIEVERS"

It was mid-morning in a well-known psychiatric hospital. The ward was quiet because most patients were away in the occupational therapy department and only those women not deemed fit to leave the ward remained. A nurse was helping a patient who was having difficulty weaving a basket. Another patient approached and said, "Nurse, there is a naked man on the fire escape." The nurse calmly asked the patient if she had seen one and continued with what she was doing. Hallucinations and delusions were common on that ward. Again the patient approached her, this time the response was some non-committal phrase not exactly contradicting the statement but not agreeing with it either. On the third approach the patient pleaded, "Come and see".

Sure enough when they looked out together at the fire escape there was a man completely devoid of any clothing or any other cover for that matter. It was not what the nurse's training and experience so far had led her to expect. To her mind it would have been almost certain that the patient was deluded or hallucinating. But despite her doubts there was a naked man on the fire escape. I repeat there WAS a naked man on the fire escape.

IF YOU HAVE FINISHED WITH THIS BOOK
PASS IT ON TO SOMEONE ELSE WHO MAY BE
INTERESTED – EITHER DIRECTLY OR BY
DONATING IT TO A BOOK SALE
OR CHARITY SHOP.

THANK YOU.

# FURTHER READING

*Multiple Chemical Sensitivity – A Survival Guide*
Pamela Reed Gibson
(New Harbinger Publications, 1999)

*Chemical Sensitivity and the Allergic Response*
William J., Rea MD
Ear, Nose and Throat Journal, Vol 67, No 1, (January 1988)
(Little, Brown and Company, Boston, MA.)

*The Complete Guide to Food Allergy and Intolerance*
Professor Jonathan Brostoff and Linda Gamlin
(Bloomsbury, 1989 [1998 paperback])
This has a useful section on chemical sensitivity.

*Not All in the Mind*
Dr Richard Mackarness
(Pan Books, 1976)
ISBN 0 330 24592 9

*Chemical Victims*
Dr Richard Mackarness
(Pan Books, 1980)
ISBN 0 33025937

*Pure White and Deadly – How Sugar is Killing Us and What We Can Do To Stop It*
John Yudkin
with new Introduction by Robert H. Lustig MD (2012)
(Penguin Books, 1972, 1986, 2012)
ISBN 978-0-241-96528-3

*Silent Spring*
Rachel Carson
(Penguin Books, 1962)
ISBN 13:978-0141-18494-4

Leaflets and newsletters from *Allergy UK* when it had a "Chemical Sensitivity" section.

# USEFUL ADDRESSES

Action Against Allergy
PO Box 278
Twickenham TW1 4QQ
t. 0208 892 2711/4949
AAA@actionagainstallergy.freeserve.co.uk
www.actionagainstallergy.co.uk

Action for ME
www.actionforme.org.uk

Allergy UK Helpline
t. 01322 619898
www.allergyuk.org

E. cloth System Environmental Products
The Brewery
Bells Yew Green
Tunbridge Wells
Kent TN3 9BD
t. 01892 752199
info@enviroproducts.co.uk
www.e-cloth.com

ECOS Organic Paints
Unit 19, Heysham Business Park
Middleton Road
Heysham
Lancs LA3 3PP
t. 01524 852371

Electro Sensitivity UK
BM Box ES-UK
London WC1N 3XX
t. 0845 643 9748
Enquirers@es-uk.info
www.es-uk-info

EnviroVent
EnviroVent House
Hornbeam Business Park
Harrogate
North Yorkshire
t.0845 2727807
www.homeventilation.co.uk
enquiries@envirovent.co.uk

(Single fans to whole house ventilation systems resulting in cleaner air supply, cutting down on VOCs and preventing condensation and moulds.)

The Healthy House Limited
t. 0845 450 5950 or 01453 752216
www.healthy-house.co.uk

(provides a wide range of products suitable for those with allergies and sensitivities.)

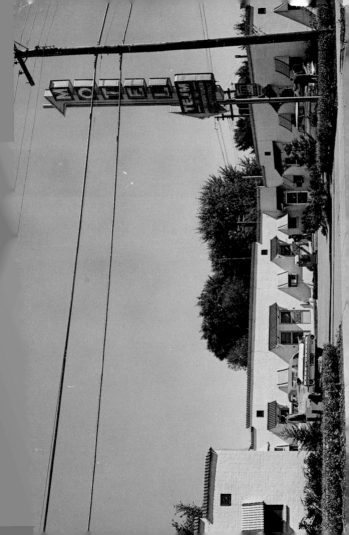

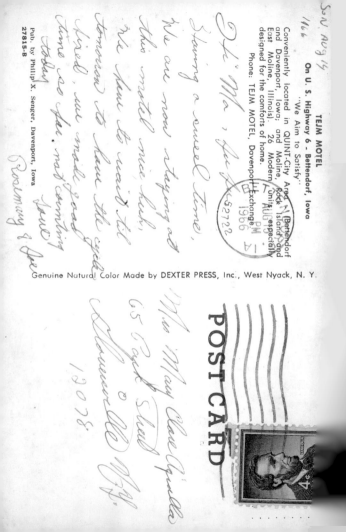

TEIM MOTEL

On U.S. Highway 6 - Bettendorf, Iowa

"We Aim to Satisfy"

Conveniently located in QUINT-City Area, (Bettendorf and Davenport, Iowa; and Moline, Rock Island and East Moline, Illinois). 26 Modern Units, especially designed for the comforts of home.

Phone: TEIM MOTEL, Davenport Exchange.

Pub. by Philip X. Senger, Davenport, Iowa

27815-B

POST CARD

The Laundry Labs at Green Line Products Ltd
Control House
Station Road
Radlett
Herts WD7 8JY
t. +44 84 5404 9525
Info@dryerballs.eu

(Dryerballs can be obtained at supermarkets and other outlets.)

ME Association
www.meassociation.orguk

Identity tags:
The Medical Alert Foundation
327-329 Upper Fourth Street
Milton Keynes  MK9 1EH
t. 0800 581420
Info@medicalalert.org.uk
www.medicalalert.org.uk

Universal Medical ID
t. 0800 0556504
www.universalmedicalid.co.uk

SOS talisman from H Samuel

# GLOSSARY

Anaphylaxis – a serious allergic condition of rapid onset that might be fatal

Biocide – chemical or micro-organism which can deter, make harmless or have controlling effect on a harmful organism

Candida – yeast-like fungi which are normal in the human bowel but can cause problems if they settle in other parts of the body. It is believed that if they increase to become disproportionate to other micro-organisms in the bowel they cause health problems. Research is being done as to the normal balance of gut organisms

Carcinogenic – causing cancer

Central nervous system – the brain, spinal cord and nerves that leave it

Chlorofluocarbons – man-made compounds containing chlorine, fluorine and carbon. Totally artificial, first made in the 1930s

Cognitive function – awareness, perception and memory

Desensitisation – a treatment aimed at stopping an individual being sensitive or allergic to something specific by introducing a weakened form of the substance they are sensitive to often in the form of an injection. It can be a dangerous procedure and needs to be performed in a place where good emergency care will be immediately available

Detoxification pathways – means by which body combats substances it finds harmful to it

Ecosystem – a community of living organisms, plants and microbes

Emission – something given off or out such as a gas or a light

Endocrine system – the glands which produce secretions which pass straight into the blood and affect distant parts of the body

Enzyme – substance produced by body cells that cause changes within the body

Fibromyalgia – chronic disease in which pain in many parts of the body is the main feature but with similarities to Myalgic Encephalomyelitis

Foetus – unborn animal including the human baby

Gas – something in an air-like state. Usually invisible, it does not become liquid or solid at normal temperatures, cf. Vapour

Gastro-intestinal – to do with the digestive organs

Herbicide – weed killer

Idiopathic – arising without recognisable cause, or of spontaneous origin

Immune system – this protects the body from disease, usually from infections

Incitant – that which stimulates something to happen. In this context whatever causes symptoms to occur

Ingest – taking material into the gastro-intestinal tract

Insecticide – chemical used to kill insects

Leaching – drawing out of a substance from a mixture

Leviathan – sea monster mentioned in the Bible

Malignancy – here means cancer

Mau Mau – revolutionaries in Kenya between1952 and 1960

Migraine – recurrent headache with nausea, vomiting and sensitivity to light

Myalgic encephalomyelitis – chronic disease with fatigue, pain and memory problems

Nasal – to do with the nose

Oestrogen – a female hormone

Peak flow – the maximum speed of breathing

Physiological – to do with the function of living systems, e.g. the human body

Porphyria – unpleasant disease causing acute abdominal pain and symptoms of the nervous system

Proliferation – increase, spread

Protein – important component of the body. In the diet protein is obtained from meat, fish, peas, beans and others

Psychogenic – physical disease stemming from emotional or mental stresses

Psychological – to do with the mind and its function

Respiratory – to do with breathing

Retina – light-sensitive area at the back of the eyeball

Sigmund Freud – Austrian doctor known as the father of psychoanalysis. He became a major influence on twentieth century thought

Smog – fog that has been intensified by smoke and other pollutants

Solvent – substance which dissolves others

Stressor – something of any kind that causes stress to an organism

Symptom – something not normal about the body of which the patient is aware

Traumatised – damaged. Originally trauma meant physical damage. Commonly now it means emotional damage

Vaccine – preparation of dead or living micro-organisms used to treat or prevent disease

Vapour – state of a solid or liquid which has gone into the air in the form of a gas

Ventilate – cause air to circulate

# HANDBOOK INDEX

Activate carbon 99, 104

Additives 109

Adhesives 47

Advocate (see Articulate advocate)

Aftershave 4

Air conditioning 9, 132, 133

Air freshener 12, 28, 48, 57, 60, 73, 128

Air pollution 28, 29, 35, 39, 126-7, (see also pollutant, pollution)

Air purifier 99

Aluminium 37, 118, 119

Amalgam (see Dental amalgam)

Ammonia 8

Anaesthetic 55

Anaphylaxis 20, 30, 56

Anti-candida diet 124

Antifreeze 43

Antihistamine 22

Antiseptics 25

Anxiety 19, 66

Arsenic 33

Arthritis 17, 57

Articulate advocate 78, 131, 136

Asbestos 36

Asthma 17, 19, 26, 37, 38, 51, 53, 67

Background pollution 4, 47, 48

Bacteria (see micro-organisms)

Baking soda (see Sodium bicarbonate)

Bees 40

Benzene 43

Biocide 26

Bloating, Bloatedness 19, 123

Bonaparte, Napoleon 33

Books 104

Borax 92, 94, 100

Brain fog 4, 8, 19, 73, 77, 124
Bronopol 27
Calcium 114, 139
Camelford 37
Campaign for Real Ale 123
Candida 9, 57, 68-70, 123-124
Cars 9, 26, 104
Chemotherapy 55
Chlorine 57
Chlorophyll 112
Cholesterol 115,116
Cigarette smoke 10, 27, 56, 130
Clothing 61, 103
Cloves 115
Coal 35
Concentration 19
Cosmetics 27, 87
Crematoria 42
Darwin, Charles 34
Dental amalgam 42, 68
Dentist 52, 69, 107, 135
Deodorant 4
Depression 19, 22
Desensitisation 22
Detergent 5, 6, 47, 129
Detoxification pathways 10
Diarrhoea 29

Diesel 37
Dietician 108
Dioxin 44, 47, 121
Disbeliever 4, 11, 146
Dishcloth 90
Disinfectant 25, 26, 27
Disseminator 4,130, 131, 137
Dissociation 66, 67
Doctors 13-16, 21, 23-24, 52-55, 62-3, 66, 126, 135
Dry cleaning 95
Earache 29
Ear, nose and throat 19
Eczema 34, 51
Egyptians, ancient 32
Endocrine system 9
Enzymes 10
EpiPen 56
Exhaustion 19
Extractor fan 97, 99
Fabric conditioner 5, 47
Fainting 19
Fatigue 8, 19, 44, 69, 70
Fibromyalgia 9
Fire retardants 51
Fish 47
Flu 8, 20, 69, 78, 106
Fog 35

Food chain 47

Food containers, wrappers 45-46, 118

Formaldehyde 26, 29, 40, 43

Freud, Sigmund 14

Friars balsam (see Tincure of benzoin co)

Fruit 22, 113

Furnishings 62,

Garlic 115

General practitioner (see Doctors)

George III 33

Germs (see Micro-organisms)

Glossy paper 104

Gluten intolerance 52

Gut dysbiosis 124

Hand washing 78, 105

Hay fever 11, 38

Headache 6,19, 44, 53, 69

Health professionals 2-3, 12, 14-16, 21-23, 75, 78-79, 80,108, 136

Herbicide 25, 47

Hospital 23, 28-29, 54-56, 63

Incitant 5, 9, 12, 18, 21, 23, 26, 59, 71-72, 77, 79, 108, 139

Indoor pollution 48

Inhaler 125

Inks 47

Insecticide 40, 47

Insomnia 19, 122, 138

Interstitial cystitis 17

Iodine 115

Irritability 19

Kohl 32

Lactose intolerance 52

Laundry 54

Laxatives 22, 47

Lead 11, 31, 47

Lethargy 8, 19, 69-70, 124

Light headedness 19

Lung rot 32

Lupus 17

Magazines 104

Magnesium 22

Marmalade 6

Masks (see Vapour masks)

Mau Mau 10

Medium Density Fibreboard 26

Menthol 125

Mercury 33, 42, 69

Mesothelioma 36

Methanol 27

Microfibre 89

Micro-organisms 77, 90, 105

Migraine 15, 17, 42, 66-69
Moths 95
Mould 95
Multiple Sclerosis 17
Myalgic encephalomyelitis 9, 17, 52, 53, 61
Nasal (see nose)
Nausea 19, 44
Nitric oxide 17, 22
Nose 19, 125
Outgas 5, 95, 103
Oven 54
Ozone 29, 37, 39, 127, 141
Pain 19
Paint 6, 25, 44, 47, 55, 57, 82, 100
Parfum (see perfume)
Parkinson's disease 17, 41
Pass out 5, 73
Perfume 4, 5, 8, 12, 14, 15, 25, 30, 45, 53-57, 60, 84, 88, 105
Pesticide 25, 41, 117, 127
Photocopiers 40
Phthalates 45
Plastic 60, 118
Polish 8
Pollutant, Pollution 9, 26, 28, 35, 40, 42, 47, 48, 64, 67, 102, 112, 126, 144

Polychlorinated biphenyls 44, 121
Polyethylene terephthalate ethylene (PETE) 46
Polythene 118
Porphyria 9, 33
Preservative 109
Protocol 14, 23
Psychiatric symptoms 16, 19
Psychological 12-14, 72
Pyrethroid 60
Radiotherapy 55
Rhinitis 13
Rubber gloves 90
Sea kelp 115
Shampoo 27, 47, 86
Shoes 82
Shower head 96
Skin 19
Sleep,
    irresistible 19
    lack of 53
Smog 35, 38
Soap 15, 78, 106
Sodium bicarbonate 84, 91-94
Sodium lauryl sulphate 51
Spheroidal Carbonacous Particles 35
Spices 56

Steam cleaners 89

Sunscreen 87

Surfactant 47

Swimming 127

Symptoms of MCS 8, 58, 72

Talcum powder 86

Terpenes 43

Tincture of benzoin co 125

Tiredness (see Fatigue)

Toilet preparations 5, 10, 16, 25-27, 46, 48, 84

Toothpaste 47

Ulcerative colitis 17

Urea formaldehyde foam 27

Vacuum cleaner 91, 97

Value Added Tax xiii

Vapour masks 24, 79, 80

Vaseline petroleum jelly 81

Vehicle exhaust emissions 4, 16, 25, 34, 37, 53, 64, 67, 102

Ventilation, ventilators 48-49, 59, 97-100

Vicks 126

Vinegar 91-96

Vitamins 22, 111, 120

Wallpaper 34

Washing up liquid 93

Weakness 19

Whiteboard markers 72

Wood preserver 25, 57

Zinc 6